due may 30/12

D0047488

RAW AND BEYOND

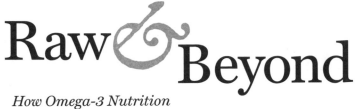

Raw & Beyond

How Omega-3 Nutrition

Is Transforming the Raw Food Paradigm

VICTORIA BOUTENKO

ELAINA LOVE

CHAD SARNO

North Atlantic Books
Berkeley, California

Published by
North Atlantic Books
P.O. Box 12327
Berkeley, California 94712

Cover photo © istockphoto.com/vm and istockphoto.com/Vitalina Rybakova
Cover and book design by Claudia Smelser
Printed in the United States of America

Raw and Beyond is sponsored by the Society for the Study of Native Arts and
Sciences, a nonprofit educational corporation whose goals are to develop an
educational and cross-cultural perspective linking various scientific, social, and
artistic fields; to nurture a holistic view of arts, sciences, humanities, and healing; and to publish and distribute literature on the relationship of mind, body,
and nature.

North Atlantic Books' publications are available through most bookstores. For
further information, visit our website at www.northatlanticbooks.com or call
800-733-3000.

MEDICAL DISCLAIMER: The following information is intended for general
information purposes only. Individuals should always see their health care pro-
vider before administering any suggestions made in this book. Any application
of the material set forth in the following pages is at the reader's discretion and
is his or her sole responsibility.

LIBRARY OF CONGRESS CATALOGING-IN-PUBLICATION DATA

Boutenko, Victoria.
  Raw and beyond : how omega-3 nutrition is transforming the raw food
paradigm / Victoria Boutenko, Elaina Love, and Chad Sarno.
      p. cm.
  Includes bibliographical references and index.
  ISBN 978-1-58394-357-1
1. Raw food diet. 2. Vegetarian cooking. 3. High-omega-3 fatty acid
diet—Recipes. I. Love, Elaina. II. Sarno, Chad. III. Title.
  RM237.5.B6925 2011
  613.263—dc23   2011036659

1 2 3 4 5 6 7 8 9   United   16 15 14 13 12 11

Printed on recycled paper

We dedicate this book to Cherie Soria,
master chef and inspiration to us all.

CONTENTS

A Note from the Authors   ix

PART ONE *Three Stories of Raw Transformation*   1

     Victoria Boutenko   3

     Elaina Love   23

     Chad Sarno   31

PART TWO *Recipes*   37

     Appetizers, Antipasti, and Finger Foods   39

     Salads   51

     Dressings   69

     Soups   77

     Breads, Crackers, and Chips   93

     Entrées   103

     Desserts   119

     Drinks   133

Acknowledgments   147

Index   149

About the Authors   157

A NOTE FROM THE AUTHORS

In this book we present our revised approach to raw food. All three of us discovered the benefits of eating raw at about the same time, some sixteen years ago. Throughout this period, we often participated in the same events, either serving raw food or teaching others how to prepare it. In 2010, our paths crossed again at a Living Light Culinary Arts Institute in California. We were intrigued that we had all independently come to similar conclusions about our diets and had begun practicing "beyond raw" cuisine. As we discussed this coincidence, we decided it was important to share our adjusted raw food diet with our followers.

PART ONE

Three Stories of Raw Transformation

VICTORIA BOUTENKO

TWO MAJOR MISTAKES I MADE
IN MY RAW FOOD DIET

A life spent making mistakes is not only more honorable, but more useful than a life spent doing nothing. —GEORGE BERNARD SHAW

For the last nineteen years I have been a raw food pioneer, and as a pioneer I recognize the mistakes I've made as well as the successes I've had on this path.

I became interested in the raw food diet in 1993. As there were very few books about raw food at that time, I was able to read most of them within a couple of months. I became especially inspired after reading *Raw Eating* by A. T. Hovannessian and *Enzyme Nutrition* by Edward Howell. The latter book I read aloud to my family. I became convinced that the raw food diet was the most natural diet for all creatures in the world, including humans.

In his book, Dr. Howell advised readers to consume a diet as high in raw food as possible. I was so motivated by Howell's research, and my family was so in need of healing beyond what the medical establishment could offer us, that in January 1994 I put my whole family on a 100 percent raw food diet.

Today, eighteen years later, I still wholeheartedly appreciate that decision. I believe that it saved my life and healed such serious illnesses in my family as arrhythmia, diabetes, rheumatoid arthritis, and asthma. I won't repeat my family story here as it can be found in all of my books and on the internet. Rather, I would like to discuss the mistakes I made in my raw food journey and how I corrected them. I view my family's eighteen years of eating raw as an opportunity to present the raw food diet to others in a more practical way.

For many years the theory of the raw food diet seemed so flawless to me that I couldn't find any errors in it. I was following a 100 percent raw food lifestyle and was trying to inspire as many others as possible to follow. Years later, to my surprise, I found major flaws hiding in two of my favorite statements:

"Anything raw is superior to anything cooked."

"Raw food is best for humans because all animals in the world consume 100 percent raw food."

Anything raw is superior to anything cooked. For a long time, this conclusion seemed clear and obvious to me. Yet this statement is correct only when we compare the nutritional value of the same foods in their raw form versus their cooked form—a raw cabbage to cooked cabbage, raw potato to fried potato, raw walnut to roasted walnut, and so on. I never bothered to investigate if there was any cooked food that had more nutritional value than any raw food. For example, what is more nourishing, steamed asparagus or cashew nuts? Lightly cooked red cabbage or an ounce of raw almond butter? A baked apple or a slice of a raw cake? If I had posed these questions, the answers would have proven the statement "Anything raw is superior to anything cooked" false.

Countless variations of cooked food exist in the world, depending on different cooking methods, ethnic customs, and choices of local foods. The nutritional value of cooked food depends on the time and intensity of the cooking process. Generally, the lighter the cooking, the higher the nutritional value of a food will be. For example, steamed or lightly cooked vegetables can retain up to 80 percent of their vitamins,[1] minerals, and other nutrients, while deep-fried, roasted, or smoked vegetables lose most of their nutritional value and also gain toxic components such as acrylamides, carcinogens, mutagens, and others.

Raw food is best for humans because all animals in the world consume 100 percent raw food. This was another main argument I used in favor of the raw food diet. I didn't pay attention to the fact that most animals (excluding carnivores, which devour large quantities of meat all at once) must eat for at least six hours a day in order to get enough nutrition in their diets.

Over the years, these flaws in my thinking began to reveal themselves as my family experienced different reactions to eating raw. The first signs of imperfect health appeared after approximately seven years on a 100 percent raw food diet. At first, everyone in my family began to notice small symptoms such as a wart on a hand or a gray hair. My skin became very dry. Later these symptoms increased, and along with strong unhealthy cravings raised questions about the completeness of the raw food diet in its existing form.

---

1. *Journal of the Science of Food and Agriculture,* November 2003.

ESSENTIAL CHANGES WE MADE
TO OUR RAW FOOD PLAN
Green Smoothies

Usually books about the raw food diet direct people to eat mostly raw fruits, vegetables, nuts, and seeds. That's what we did, but obviously something was missing in that combination.

Motivated by my family's increase in unhealthy symptoms, I started new research that led me to discover the exceptionally high nutritional value of greens. (By greens, I mean the leafy green parts of plants that can be folded around a finger.) Greens are the only living thing in the world that can transform sunshine into food that all creatures can consume. Chlorophyll is a miraculous substance, as it is in essence liquefied sunshine.

Green leaves are vital for the survival of all living beings on our planet, including humans. In fact, green leaves are as essential to human existence as water, air, and sunlight. I have conducted a lot of research and found that the nutritional composition of greens matches human nutritional needs to an amazing degree. Greens contain most of the essential minerals, vitamins, and even amino acids that humans need for optimal health. You can find more information about the nutritional value of greens in my books *Green for Life* and *Green Smoothie Revolution*.

The problem was that my family members, myself included, didn't like the taste of greens and were not accustomed to eating a lot of them. In an attempt to find the best way to consume more greens, I came up with the idea of green smoothies in September 2004. A green smoothie is a blended drink prepared with greens, ripe organic fruit, and water. Fruit camouflages the taste of greens, which helps people consume more of this valuable food in a palatable way. When blended, the nutrients from greens are absorbed more efficiently and provide many times more nutrients than other foods do, even salads. In a short time, people can get as much nutrition from green smoothies as animals get in six or more hours of eating, which is essential in our fast-paced modern lives.

The green smoothie discovery reversed many signs of health decline in my family, such as tooth sensitivity, brittle nails, hair loss, skin dryness, etc. Yet adding green smoothies to our diet still did not bring us perfect health. For example, I could not return to my ideal weight. We all had a strong feeling that something was still missing in our diet. I shared my concerns with many other raw food teachers who had maintained an all-raw diet for years, and they too agreed that something seemed lacking in their diets. My friends were constantly trying to solve their problems by taking a variety of nutritional supplements.

Omega-3s

In 2010, I became aware of the serious deficiency of omega-3 fatty acids in our diets. As soon as I read several scientific articles on the importance of omega-3s, I felt that I had arrived at an explanation for the questions I had been struggling with concerning the 100 percent raw diet. What I discovered was shocking, and it completely changed our approach to our raw food diet.

The omega-3 deficiency, common today for most people, not just raw foodists, resulted from modern dietary changes and a lack of knowledge about the effects of essential fatty acids (EFAs) on health. The omega-3 molecule is unique in its ability to rapidly change its shape. This exceptional flexibility of omega-3s is passed to the organs that absorb it.[2] Omega-3s thin the blood of humans and animals as well as the sap of plants. As a result of these qualities, omega-3s are utilized by the fastest-functioning organs in the body. For example, omega-3s enable our hearts to beat properly, our blood to flow freely, our eyes to see, and our brains to make decisions faster and more clearly.

Omega-6 fatty acids, on the other hand, serve the opposite function: they thicken the blood of humans and animals as well as the juices of plants. Omega-6s solidify and cause inflammation of the tissues. Some scientists link an excess of omega-6s in the human diet to such conditions as heart disease, stroke, arthritis, asthma, menstrual cramps, diabetes, headaches, and tumor metastases. I would like to emphasize, however, that the omega-6 fatty acids are not "bad"; they serve an important function in the body as well, but must be consumed in a proper ratio to omega-3s.

Because the unique flexibility of the omega-3 molecule makes it highly perishable, in recent years genetic engineers have been manipulating the DNA of seeds, trying to develop strains with higher omega-6 and lower omega-3 content in order to prolong the storage life of seeds and the oils made from them. In addition, most farm animals, such as cattle, sheep, pigs, and chickens, have increasingly been fed soy, corn, and other grains instead of grass and hay, which has altered the balance of omegas present in meat. People who consume animal products would benefit from knowing that the meat from animals that consume grass is high in omega-3s while the

---

2. Susan Allport, *The Queen of Fats: Why Omega-3s Were Removed from the Western Diet and What We Can Do to Replace Them* (Berkeley: University of California Press, 2006).

meat from animals that consume corn and other grains is high in omega-6s. Even fish aren't guaranteed to be a good source of omega-3s anymore. Omega-3 fatty acids are the main reason doctors recommend eating fish regularly, but farmed fish are now fed a grain-heavy diet, vastly reducing their levels of fish oils. A very popular fish in recent years, tilapia, contains twice the level of omega-6 as omega-3. Last year, the *New York Times* reported that "compared with other fish, farmed tilapia contains relatively small amounts of beneficial omega-3 fatty acids ... because the fish are fed corn and soy instead of lake plants and algae, the diet of wild tilapia."[3]

Our modern grain- and oil-heavy diet has resulted in most people, whether vegetarians or meat-eaters, consuming way too many omega-6 fatty acids and not enough omega-3s. It turns out that the majority of Americans are seriously deficient in omega-3 essential fatty acids. According to a recent study by the Harvard School of Public Health, omega-3 deficiencies account for nearly 96,000 preventable deaths each year in the United States.[4]

In order to correct this problem, we need first to find out what the healthiest balance of essential fatty acids is. Most of the articles I have read suggest that the ratio of omega-6s to omega-3s should be 3:1 or 2:1. The typical American diet today contains anywhere from a 10:1 to a 20:1 ratio of omega-6s to omega-3s, an imbalance associated with a high rate of disease. The Institute of Medicine, the health arm of the National Academy of Sciences, recommends an intake of approximately

---

3. Elisabeth Rosenthal, "Another Side of Tilapia, the Perfect Factory Fish," *New York Times*, May 2, 2011.
4. "Omega-3 Fatty Acid Deficiency takes 96,000 Lives Annually in the US," Reuters News Service, June 25, 2009.

10:1, much higher than the ratio recommended by Sweden (5:1) or Japan (4:1). The ratio in Japan is associated with a very low incidence of heart and other disease.

We can increase our consumption of omega-3s in different ways. According to Dr. Frank Sacks, Professor of Nutrition at Harvard School of Public Health, there are two major types of omega-3 fatty acids in our diets. One type is alpha-linolenic acid (ALA), which is found in flaxseed oil, walnuts, and also in green leafy vegetables. The other type, the longer-chain fatty acids eicosapentaenoic acid (EPA) and docosahexaenoic acid (DHA), is found in fatty fish. The body partially converts ALA to EPA and DHA.

Fortunately, omega-3 is widely available in all greens, especially in spinach, romaine, and arugula. One of the highest levels of omega-3s can be found in purslane, a widespread wild green. Green smoothies are an ideal way to increase one's intake of these beneficial omega-3 fatty acids and thus work toward overcoming a wide variety of health conditions. At the same time, to further reduce omega-6s, people can decrease their consumption of nuts.

The following list of ratios of omega-3s to omega-6s will help you see which common raw foods to eat more of if you wish to boost your omega-3 fatty acid intake.

RATIO OF OMEGA-3s TO OMEGA-6s IN OILS, SEEDS, AND GREENS

Flaxseed oil: (1 tablespoon)
Total omega-3 fatty acids   7,196 mg (4.2 times more omega-3s)
Total omega-6 fatty acids   1,715 mg
http://nutritiondata.self.com/facts/fats-and-oils/7554/2

Hempseed oil: (1 tablespoon)

Total omega-3 fatty acids   3,000 mg

Total omega-6 fatty acids   8,000 mg (2.7 times more omega-6s)

http://hempbasics.com/shop/cms-display/hemp-seed-nutrition.html

Sunflower oil: (1 tablespoon)

Total omega-3 fatty acids   5.0 mg

Total omega-6 fatty acids   3,905 mg (781 times more omega-6s)

http://nutritiondata.self.com/facts/fats-and-oils/7945/2

Safflower oil: (1 tablespoon)

Total omega-3 fatty acids   0 mg

Total omega-6 fatty acids   10,073 mg (too many! omega-6s)

http://nutritiondata.self.com/facts/fats-and-oils/573/2

Sesame oil: (1 tablespoon)

Total omega-3 fatty acids   40.5 mg

Total omega-6 fatty acids   5,576 mg (138 times more omega-6s)

http://nutritiondata.self.com/facts/fats-and-oils/511/2

Corn oil: (1 tablespoon)

Total omega-3 fatty acids   157 mg

Total omega-6 fatty acids   7,224 mg (46 times more omega-6s)

http://nutritiondata.self.com/facts/fats-and-oils/580/2

Canola oil: (1 tablespoon)

Total omega-3 fatty acids   1,031 mg

Total omega-6 fatty acids   2,532 mg (2.5 times more omega-6s)

http://nutritiondata.self.com/facts/fats-and-oils/7947/2

Olive oil: (1 tablespoon)

Total omega-3 fatty acids   103 mg

Total omega-6 fatty acids   1,318 mg (13 times more omega-6s)

http://nutritiondata.self.com/facts/fats-and-oils/509/2

Cocoa butter: (1 tablespoon)
Total omega-3 fatty acids   13.5 mg
Total omega-6 fatty acids   378 mg (28 times more omega-6s)
http://nutritiondata.self.com/facts/fats-and-oils/570/2

Coconut oil: (1 tablespoon)
Total omega-3 fatty acids   0 mg
Total omega-6 fatty acids   243 mg (only omega-6s)
http://nutritiondata.self.com/facts/fats-and-oils/508/2

Coconut (shredded, dry) meat, raw: (1 cup)
Total omega-3 fatty acids   0 mg
Total omega-6 fatty acids   293 mg (only omega-6s)
http://nutritiondata.self.com/facts/nut-and-seed-products/3106/2

Avocado, raw, puréed: (1 cup)
Total omega-3 fatty acids   253 mg
Total omega-6 fatty acids   3,886 mg (15 times more omega-6s)
http://nutritiondata.self.com/facts/fruits-and-fruit-juices/1844/2

Chia seeds: (100 g)
Total omega-3 fatty acids   17,552 mg (3 times more omega-3s)
Total omega-6 fatty acids   5,785 mg
http://nutritiondata.self.com/facts/nut-and-seed-products/3061/2

Flaxseeds: (100 g)
Total omega-3 fatty acids   22,813 mg (3.9 times more omega-3s)
Total omega-6 fatty acids   5,911 mg
http://nutritiondata.self.com/facts/nut-and-seed-products/3163/2

Hempseeds: (100 g)
Total omega-3 fatty acids   7,740 mg
Total omega-6 fatty acids   19,360 mg (2.5 times more omega-6s)
http://en.wikipedia.org/wiki/Hemp

Sunflower seeds: (1 cup)

Total omega-3 fatty acids   34.0 mg

Total omega-6 fatty acids   10,602 mg (312 times more omega-6s)

http://nutritiondata.self.com/facts/nut-and-seed-products/3076/2

Sesame seeds: (1 cup)

Total omega-3 fatty acids   541 mg

Total omega-6 fatty acids   30,776 mg (57 times more omega-6s)

http://nutritiondata.self.com/facts/nut-and-seed-products/3070/2

Pumpkin seeds: (1 cup)

Total omega-3 fatty acids   250 mg

Total omega-6 fatty acids   28,571 mg (114 times more omega-6s)

http://nutritiondata.self.com/facts/nut-and-seed-products/3066/2

Walnuts: (1 cup)

Total omega-3 fatty acids   10,623 mg

Total omega-6 fatty acids   44,567 mg (4.2 times more omega-6s)

http://nutritiondata.self.com/facts/nut-and-seed-products/3138/2

Almonds: (1 cup)

Total omega-3 fatty acids   5.7 mg

Total omega-6 fatty acids   11,462 mg (2,011 times more omega-6s)

http://nutritiondata.self.com/facts/nut-and-seed-products/3085/2

Cashews: (1 cup)

Total omega-3 fatty acids   62.0 mg

Total omega-6 fatty acids   7,782 mg (126 times more omega-6s)

http://nutritiondata.self.com/facts/nut-and-seed-products/3095/2

Macadamia nuts, raw: (1 cup)

Total omega-3 fatty acids   276 mg

Total omega-6 fatty acids   1,737 mg (6.3 times more omega-6s)

http://nutritiondata.self.com/facts/nut-and-seed-products/3123/2

Filberts (Hazelnuts): (1 cup)
Total omega-3 fatty acids   100 mg
Total omega-6 fatty acids   9,007 mg (90 times more omega-6s)
http://nutritiondata.self.com/facts/nut-and-seed-products/3116/2

Pine nuts: (1 cup)
Total omega-3 fatty acids   151.0 mg
Total omega-6 fatty acids   45,369 mg (300 times more omega-6s)
http://nutritiondata.self.com/facts/nut-and-seed-products/3133/2

Peanuts: (1 cup)
Total omega-3 fatty acids   4.4 mg
Total omega-6 fatty acids   22,711 mg (5,162 times more omega-6s)
http://nutritiondata.self.com/facts/legumes-and-legume-products/4355/2

Pecans: (1 cup)
Total omega-3 fatty acids   1,075 mg
Total omega-6 fatty acids   22,487 mg (21 times more omega-6s)
http://nutritiondata.self.com/facts/nut-and-seed-products/3129/2

Wheat: (1 cup)
Total omega-3 fatty acids   52 mg
Total omega-6 fatty acids   1,152 mg (22 times more omega-6s)
http://nutritiondata.self.com/facts/cereal-grains-and-pasta/5737/2

Rye: (1 cup)
Total omega-3 fatty acids   265 mg
Total omega-6 fatty acids   1,619 mg (6 times more omega-6s)
http://nutritiondata.self.com/facts/cereal-grains-and-pasta/5727/2

Oats: (1 cup)
Total omega-3 fatty acids   173 mg
Total omega-6 fatty acids   3,781 mg (22 times more omega-6s)
http://nutritiondata.self.com/facts/cereal-grains-and-pasta/5708/2

Quinoa: (1 cup)

Total omega-3 fatty acids   522 mg

Total omega-6 fatty acids   5,061 mg (10 times more omega-6s)

http://nutritiondata.self.com/facts/cereal-grains-and-pasta/5705/2

Lentils: (1 cup)

Total omega-3 fatty acids   209 mg

Total omega-6 fatty acids   776 mg (3.7 times more omega-6s)

http://nutritiondata.self.com/facts/legumes-and-legume
   -products/4337/2

Beans, snap, green, raw: (1 cup)

Total omega-3 fatty acids   39.6 mg (1.6 times more omega-3s)

Total omega-6 fatty acids   25.3 mg

http://nutritiondata.self.com/facts/vegetables-and-vegetable
   -products/2341/2

Kidney beans, boiled: (1 cup)

Total omega-3 fatty acids   301 mg (1.6 times more omega-3s)

Total omega-6 fatty acids   191 mg

http://nutritiondata.self.com/facts/legumes-and-legume
   -products/4297/2

Chickpeas, raw: (1 cup)

Total omega-3 fatty acids   202 mg

Total omega-6 fatty acids   5,186 mg (26 times more omega-6s)

http://nutritiondata.self.com/facts/legumes-and-legume
   -products/4325/2

Green peas, raw: (1 cup)

Total omega-3 fatty acids   50.8 mg

Total omega-6 fatty acids   220 mg (4.3 times more omega-6s)

http://nutritiondata.self.com/facts/vegetables-and-vegetable
   -products/2520/2

Sugar snap peas, raw: (1 cup)

Total omega-3 fatty acids   12.7 mg

Total omega-6 fatty acids   73.5 mg (5.8 times more omega-6s)

http://nutritiondata.self.com/facts/vegetables-and-vegetable
-products/2516/2

Lettuce, green leaf, raw: (1 head, 360 g)

Total omega-3 fatty acids   209 mg (2.4 times more omega-3s)

Total omega-6 fatty acids   86.4 mg

http://nutritiondata.self.com/facts/vegetables-and-vegetable
-products/2477/2

Lettuce, cos or romaine, raw: (1 head, 626 g)

Total omega-3 fatty acids   707 mg (2.4 times more omega-3s)

Total omega-6 fatty acids   294 mg

http://nutritiondata.self.com/facts/vegetables-and-vegetable
-products/2475/2

Spinach, raw: (1 bunch, 340 g)

Total omega-3 fatty acids   469 mg (5.3 times more omega-3s)

Total omega-6 fatty acids   88.4 mg

http://nutritiondata.self.com/facts/vegetables-and-vegetable
-products/2626/2

Dandelion greens, raw: (100 g)

Total omega-3 fatty acids   44 mg

Total omega-6 fatty acids   261 mg (5.9 times more omega-6s)

http://nutritiondata.self.com/facts/vegetables-and-vegetable
-products/2441/2

Arugula, raw: (100 g)

Total omega-3 fatty acids   170 mg (1.3 times more omega-3s)

Total omega-6 fatty acids   130 mg

http://nutritiondata.self.com/facts/vegetables-and-vegetable
-products/3025/2

Apples, raw: (1 medium size)
Total omega-3 fatty acids   16.4 mg
Total omega-6 fatty acids   78.3 mg (4.8 times more omega-6s)
http://nutritiondata.self.com/facts/fruits-and-fruit-juices/1809/2

Bananas, raw: (1 medium size)
Total omega-3 fatty acids   31.9 mg
Total omega-6 fatty acids   54.3 mg (1.7 times more omega-6s)
http://nutritiondata.self.com/facts/fruits-and-fruit-juices/1846/2

Strawberries, raw: (100 g)
Total omega-3 fatty acids   65.0 mg
Total omega-6 fatty acids   90.0 mg (1.4 times more omega-6s)
http://nutritiondata.self.com/facts/fruits-and-fruit-juices/2064/2

Carrots, raw: (100 g)
Total omega-3 fatty acids   2.0 mg
Total omega-6 fatty acids   115 mg (58 times more omega-6s)
http://nutritiondata.self.com/facts/vegetables-and-vegetable
  -products/2383/2

HOW OMEGA-3 NUTRITION IS TRANSFORMING THE RAW FOOD PARADIGM

When people start out on a raw food diet, many of them commonly turn to oils, nuts, and seeds to help increase their calorie intake and add a variety of fats to the fruits and vegetables they are eating. Many raw foodists create an assortment of gourmet dishes designed to replace the heavier meats and starches to which they have been accustomed on the standard American diet. That is where the problem starts. A diet rich in nuts and seeds and low in greens, fresh fruits, and vegetables inevitably leads to nutritional deficiencies, including a lack of omega-3s and overconsumption of omega-6s. These imbalances can lead to inflammation, candida, diabetes, and even obesity, the very conditions that many people are trying to avoid by adopting a raw food lifestyle in the first place.

Sooner or later, most raw foodists notice that a diet rich in nuts doesn't work. Then, after trying to sustain a raw food diet without nuts, many of them go back to some cooked food, while others look for different ways to sustain a 100 percent raw food diet.

Being 100 percent raw is a much easier task for those who live in warmer climates, because they have access to ripe, local produce year-round. In colder climates, most produce has to be delivered from far away, resulting in wilted vegetables and unripe fruits. Lack of quality produce makes sustaining a 100 percent raw diet a lot more challenging. I still don't know if it was a coincidence that my family first began to experience difficulties on a raw food diet after we moved from sunny Colorado to rainy Oregon. I think we would have avoided many of our health problems if we had included some cooked food in our diets right then, instead of loading on nuts and nut butters for several years. But "better late than never," as they say, and "everything happens for a reason"—now everyone in my family has acquired knowledge that has enabled us to correct our eating patterns. The best outcome is that we are sharing our valuable experience with other people, helping them to avoid many painful mistakes.

New information about omegas has radically changed the foundation on which the raw food diet is based. A typical raw food meal used to consist of raw fruits, vegetables, nuts, and seeds. Many popular raw recipes, such as nut loaf, nut patties, nut burgers, cakes, and pies, contain large quantities of nuts and seeds. My family created a large number of these traditionally rich recipes ourselves, which were published in our early books and videotapes and were discontinued a couple of years ago. In our latest recipe books we have replaced nuts with grated vegetables and greens.

Nuts have long been considered a convenient source of raw nutrition as they are compact and full of calories—they are handy on their own or in energy bars as everyday snacks, for outdoor activities, and when traveling. I now understand that relying on nuts or energy bars can be unhealthy because of their high level of omega-6s. Of course, some bars can be made of seeds high in omega-3s, such as hemp, flax, walnuts, or chia, but their shelf life will be very short due to the tendency of omega-3s to quickly become rancid.

Raw foodists who want a healthy, sustainable raw food diet need to focus mostly on whole foods, salads, smoothies, and juices, with occasional tiny portions of nuts and seeds. It can be tough to maintain a 100 percent raw food diet with such restrictions. Many long-term raw foodists have already intuitively adopted this more limited version of a 100 percent raw diet, and others have shifted to a high-raw diet, adding back some cooked foods.

Elaina Love, Chad Sarno, and I have been close friends for about sixteen years. Our friendship developed on both personal and professional grounds. During these years, we went through different stages and discoveries in the raw food lifestyle almost simultaneously. When we ran into each other in busy kitchens at various retreats and festivals all over the world, we happily shared family news and exchanged our thoughts and new culinary ideas.

In 2010, we ran into each other again at the Living Light Culinary Arts Institute in Fort Bragg, California. We were impressed with and inspired by the similarities in our latest raw diet transitions. After our meeting we kept corresponding and discussing this phenomenon, and decided that now is the perfect time to share our vision of a new raw food paradigm with our followers.

This is a new kind of raw recipe book. The majority of recipes don't contain any nuts, seeds, or oils. You will find lots of soups, salads, desserts, and other dishes that come directly from our own kitchens and daily meals. Chad, Elaina, and I have been enhancing our raw recipes using a healthier ratio of omegas. Especially for this book, we have re-created several traditional raw gourmet dishes, using new ingredients to significantly reduce their omega-6 content. My daughter, Valya, learned to prepare several tasty dishes that are rich in omega-3s and are very satisfying, so I asked her to contribute twelve of her favorite recipes for this book. We have also provided several recipes that include some light cooking (these are marked by the words RAW, COOKED, or SOME COOKED). I am sure that some readers will find it a very unexpected twist that three well-known raw chefs have created a recipe book that contains some cooked foods. I, too, am shocked when I read this. Yet I hope that these recipes will improve your health, satisfy your cravings, and bring more balance into your life.

MY PRESENT DIET

You can see from the table on pages 10–17 that most nuts have an extremely high omega-6 content. For example, almonds contain two thousand times more omega-6s than omega-3s. That explains to me why after several years on a raw food diet I developed a severe dislike of most nuts. If I was given a raw treat containing nuts, I would feel very sick later, even vomit. I have heard similar stories from countless other people.

For almost seventeen years my main caloric intake came from nuts. As a 100 percent raw foodist, without nuts I could not consume the 1,600 calories per day that I needed. Some people can eat a lot of fruit. I enjoy eating my fruits daily but I am unable to get all my calories from fruit. Green smoothies work well for nutrients, but do not provide enough calories.

My experience and research has led me to a high-raw diet for a sustainable life. In 2010 I decided to remove almonds, pine nuts, cashews, nut butters, tahini, and other combinations of raw foods made with nuts, seeds, and oils from my diet. Instead, I added a small amount of steamed asparagus, broccoli, bok choy, and some other lightly cooked greens and vegetables. I now consider myself to be 90–95 percent raw. I do not eat cooked foods every day; occasionally I eat them after intensive physical activity or on a cold winter day. I still believe raw greens, fruits, and vegetables to be the most beneficial foods. On page 22 is my own food pyramid (left) for daily sustainable life.

In this pyramid, by healthy fats I mean nuts, seeds, oils, and fruit that contain a ratio of omegas beneficial for health, such as flax seeds and oil, chia seeds, hempseeds, walnuts, and others. Occasionally, I add small amounts of olive oil or avocado to my salads. While I never consume coconut oil, I love Thai (young) coconuts. I believe that without ripe organic fruit, the human diet is not complete, so I try to eat only ripe organic fruit because I am convinced that any other kind of fruit is not natural for human health.

I still believe that a 100 percent raw food diet is an effective practice as a way of natural healing. It was very beneficial for

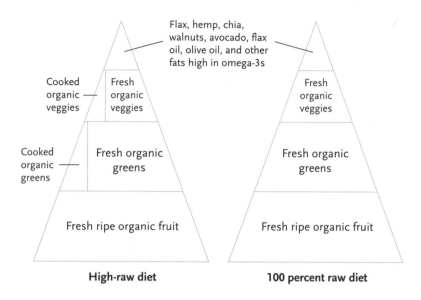

FOOD PYRAMID FOR A HIGH-RAW DIET VERSUS 100 PERCENT RAW

my family during the first years of our raw food journey. Periodically, especially after extensive traveling, I will go on a 100 percent raw food diet for several days or weeks, only now my raw food diet includes a very limited amount of healthy nuts. The pyramid on the right is my own food pyramid for healing and detoxing.

I no longer feel that anything is missing in my diet. I feel good and my weight is steadily normalizing. In addition, I have found a profound peace inside from abandoning a place of limitation and idealism. I choose to be healthy instead of being 100 percent raw. But I still believe that raw food is the most natural and ancient way of eating for humans. By explaining the pitfalls in my own raw food journey, I hope to motivate many more people to try a raw food diet.

ELAINA LOVE

Serious health challenges got me into raw foods in 1997. I had systemic candida and a lot of food allergies. I was prescribed some drugs that I wasn't interested in taking. At that time I found a book called *Cleanse and Purify Thyself* by Richard Anderson. A cleansing book that also talked about the importance of raw foods, it contained many testimonies from people who had cured themselves of diseases by eating a raw food diet. So I decided to do the cleanse and eat raw foods. In one month, after following a simple diet plan, I felt like a different person. As I continued with the raw food diet, my life kept getting better and better. Over the years, I've experimented with not eating raw and going back again—at one time I ate nothing but raw food for more than two years—and I always feel better when I'm eating a high-raw diet.

I still think that a 100 percent raw food diet is effective for cleansing and healing, and it is especially beneficial for people who have degenerative diseases, are in a lot of pain, or maybe even dying. But I have found that eating a 100 percent raw diet can sometimes be imbalancing; eating some cooked foods makes me feel more grounded and balanced. I know many people who have practiced an all-raw diet for a few months or longer and then decided to start eating some cooked food again. If they need to cleanse and purify at any time, they will go 100 percent raw for a while and eventually phase cooked foods back in. I also live on a 100 percent raw diet from time to time; it helps me feel balanced and better able to concentrate on the projects in my life.

I find it easy to eat all raw in the summertime, when the weather is hot and I am physically active. I will often eat raw food exclusively for weeks at a time, and then at some point my body starts to desire some cooked quinoa, beans, or root vegetables—foods that are a little more grounding. When I add them back in I do feel better, more grounded and healthier. So I don't believe the raw diet has to be all or nothing. I have found it more beneficial to first become familiar with a raw food diet and then start following my sense of what I need at any particular time. For example, as a woman, I'm affected by my monthly cycles, and my desires and cravings are different depending on what my body needs during the month. So I make my dietary choices season by season, month by month, or week by week, depending on what I'm desiring at any given time.

I have noticed that, for whatever reason, I often don't look as healthy while eating a 100 percent raw diet. I can't explain why. When I've added some cooked food back into my diet, people often say to me, "You look great! What are you doing?" I find it interesting that when I'm eating some cooked food instead of only raw, I get more compliments on my looks.

In my experience, raw food combined with a little cooked food is a more appealing diet for people to follow. In the past when I recommended a raw food diet, I frequently heard comments like: "Well, that's great for you, but a 100 percent raw diet is not doable for me, because I have a family," or "I'm too thin," or a hundred other reasons for why people can't manage a raw diet. I think that balance is the most important thing. For me, about 80 percent raw/20 percent cooked (or depending on the time of year, even more cooked) is a more balanced diet, and it's more doable for people to manage as a lifestyle. They can start adding more raw food into their diets and eventually find the right balance for themselves, rather than feeling pressured by the idea that they have to be 100 percent raw and that anything less is unacceptable. Let's say you are on a 100 percent raw diet and visit your family who eats a standard diet. They will probably be serving a cooked meal. If you are hungry and decide to have it, then you might later consider yourself a failure. On the other hand, if you say, "I eat a high-raw diet," and you think, *Okay, that was my 10 percent or 20 percent cooked food for the week,* then you let yourself off the hook emotionally. High-raw dieting allows you to blend in with society and your family more, and you are able to go through life more comfortably. When people are new to raw food, they often feel panic. *How do I leave the house for a meal? I don't know what to do.* Starting out high raw is much easier for the majority of people. It leaves a window for them to eat more raw food if they decide to.

I have found that our spiritual attitude is as important as, if not more important than, what we put in our mouths. How we view other people depends on how we are judging ourselves. Being very strict with myself around my diet led me to be judgmental and strict with other people and how I looked at the world; I was very isolated and excluded myself from a lot of things, including my family, because I felt that no one understood me. I discovered that being very dogmatic did not serve me well. Self-judgment and guilt can negatively impact our health, so trying to maintain a healthy diet is counterproductive if we don't feel like we're doing it "right" and beat ourselves up. I notice that people find themselves happier and more balanced if they give themselves a little more leeway. Becoming more flexible has certainly made me a happier and more balanced person.

Adding more greens to my diet has also made me much healthier. People often eat the wrong things on a raw food diet. There was a time when I was 100 percent raw but eating a lot of raw desserts and dates and sugary things, which was causing a lot of imbalance. The low-glycemic, low-sugar diet I eat now, rich in greens and with cooked foods like quinoa and beans, is a much healthier combination for me than eating 100 percent raw.

When I first went raw I ate a lot of nuts, as many new raw foodists do, to compensate for taking out wheat and dairy. So many raw recipes, such as our "bread" and "cheese" recipes, are nut-based. After a couple of years, my body became sensitive to nuts; my nose would start to run if I ate too many. Even now, my tongue will get sore really quickly if I eat too many nuts. I can still eat seeds, but I choose to avoid nuts as much as possible.

Still, I believe that raw gourmet food, which contains a lot of nuts, plays an important role in offering a healthy way of eating for many people. I am a raw gourmet chef; I teach and prepare raw gourmet food for a living. I think it is helpful to teach someone to make dishes like raw food lasagna, especially if they have wheat or dairy allergies. Many people who become vegetarians start eating way too much wheat and other grains. Raw gourmet food is important because it provides comfort and helps people transition away from high-allergy foods. Raw gourmet dishes also offer a nice alternative for people who want to serve their family something that's raw and more interesting than simple salads. Often families are more willing to accept a raw gourmet version of a food like lasagna because it is something they are familiar with.

However, I don't recommend staying on a raw gourmet diet for a long period of time. I have been consuming raw food for fourteen years, and in the beginning I ate a lot of what I consider gourmet foods. For example, I would make myself a pie and eat it for breakfast; I ate a lot of granolas and different pizzas and whatnot. Now when I keep a food diary for a week, writing down everything I eat, I notice that I tend to eat very simply, eating lots of big green salads with a drizzle of olive oil. On special occasions I still make beautiful gourmet dishes, but after all these years, I eat simply and don't feel deprived at all.

For many years I have been searching for the diet that would best fit everyone. While I haven't found one particular diet that works for every person, after traveling around the world and observing different eating patterns, I have noticed one important point: If people think that what they eat is good for them, they seem to do better than if they think that what they eat is bad for them. Some people eat 100 percent raw and seem to be doing well; some people who eat meat also seem to be doing well. Others, who like me are following an 80 percent raw/20 percent cooked diet, are doing really well. While I can't say I have found one diet that works for everyone, a high-raw diet with a lot of nutritious, alkalizing vegetables and greens (versus a raw diet loaded with dried fruits and nuts) seems to be the most beneficial of all. Most important is getting enough greens in their many forms—drinking green juices and smoothies, and eating big green salads, including greens such as kale, chard, spinach, and herbs. Most people I know love those foods. They thrive on them, and crave them the most.

When they get away from their diet they often say, "Oh, I can't wait to have more greens!"

Eating certain cooked foods can be more beneficial than eating raw foods. For instance, when 100 percent raw foodists are craving something heavy, they typically go for nuts. If they instead tried some steamed quinoa or pinto beans or red beans, which are high in omega-3s, they would feel a lot more satisfied than from eating nuts or dried fruit. Eating a lot of sweet foods like dates and sugary fruits elevates blood sugar and insulin levels, increasing the risk of diabetes and other health problems. Quinoa and beans are the two cooked foods I ate most in the past week. (Not rice, which seems to be too heavy for me even though it is gluten-free. I rarely eat rice because my body doesn't feel very good after eating it.) Every once in a while I eat a cooked sweet potato and sauté some kale with it, or steam some greens or broccoli. Broccoli is too hard to digest raw, so I prefer it steamed.

I like offering the healthiest foods to people. After discovering that many of the raw foods we commonly eat are high in omega-6s and low in omega-3s, it has become my goal to incorporate more omega-3-rich ingredients into my recipes. For example, I substituted many nuts with hempseeds, walnuts, flaxseed, and chia seeds. I am constantly looking for a balance of all the elements in the dishes I prepare. I enjoy finding new combinations and offering them to my customers; my dishes often come as a pleasing surprise both in taste and ingredients. For example, most people on a standard American diet I've talked to have never heard of chia seeds and didn't know of their outstanding health benefits, including their high omega-3 and protein content. I am glad that this book introduces people to a new way of eating that is simple, easy, and also more diverse.

Many people these days think it is normal to get sick often, four or five times a year. Some people suffer from cancer, diabetes, all kinds of diseases, and I believe that if they had more information about diet and nutrition, they would not have to suffer so much. For example, if people knew about the dangers of white sugar and its major role in destroying health, we would see a big reduction in problems with being overweight, tired, or irritable. Often when people become vegetarians and go off meat, they start eating a lot of pasta, breads, and other starches. When I went vegetarian I got sicker because of all the grains and glutens I ate. So I feel privileged to let people know there are other choices. I enjoy it when my family members and friends try raw food and say, "Wow, I feel energized! I didn't know I could feel this good just from eating this way!" It is gratifying to turn them on to the joy they can feel by adding greens and life-force into their diet.

I know a lot of people who say, "I tried eating raw but I gave it up—it didn't work for me," because they were thinking of it as an all-or-nothing diet. Yet I've never heard anyone say, "I tried adding more fruits and vegetables into my diet and it didn't work." That is why I usually tell people to try eating more fruits and vegetables. Nobody's going to fail at that. There are many experts who say negative things about raw foods, but everyone agrees that more fruits and vegetables in your diet is a good thing. We are just teaching people how to add more. Sometimes I tell my students that I'm going to trick them into eating more vegetables without their even knowing it. For example, I serve a wrap that has avocados and root vegetables in it. This dish tastes like a delicious burrito, and people don't realize that they are eating three or four different vegetables in the wrap. Kale chips are another example—they taste like potato chips and everyone thinks they're delicious.

Of course, such healthier eating strategies work best with people who have a certain frame of mind, who want to feel good. People who eat corn chips or pork rinds and think their life is fine are not going to switch over to a raw food diet yet. Not until they are tired of being sick, start searching, and discover the connection between their diet and their health will they want something better for themselves and get turned on to raw food more easily.

I am happy that this book adds more healthy foods to everyone's diet, instead of dictating an all-or-nothing approach to eating raw foods. I invite you to set yourself up for success by making one recipe a week, or a couple of recipes a week. Add more and more healthy dishes and see how you feel. Experiment! I am my own experiment. The reason I eat a high-raw diet is because I have experimented and have found that it works for me. It feels good; I have more energy and life force, I get up early and feel vibrant, and don't need coffee. I have experienced so many great benefits from eating raw that I believe if people try it, as opposed to blindly trusting any of us, they will find out for themselves that a raw food diet can work for them. You've got everything to gain. You get to have more energy because you're adding greens. You get to have more fun because you're finding that you don't need as much sleep. You enjoy your life more. You get along with people better, too. For me, eating cleansing and healing foods has been the key to finding pure joy in life.

CHAD SARNO

My first introduction to the relationship between health and diet was through asthma. Throughout my childhood and teenage years I struggled with that handicap. I was on many inhalers but they didn't improve my condition. Eventually, a friend of the family told me that staying away from dairy might help, so I stopped eating dairy and within six months I was off all my inhalers and never experienced an asthma attack again. That experience started me on the path of health.

Another main influence that led me to a raw food diet was through my spiritual exploration when I was young, looking into the Essene teachings. One day I found myself at Breitenbush Hot Springs, participating in an event given by Cherie Soria's Living Light Culinary Arts Institute. After I helped her cater the National Essene Gathering, Cherie asked me if I'd leave Breitenbush and be her staff chef. It was all very grassroots. At the time there were only three other people working at Living Light, kind of a traveling raw food circus. I joined them and was the staff chef on and off for a year or two. I jumped into preparing raw foods and my career as a chef snowballed from there.

I got into raw foods in 1996 and stayed on a 100 percent raw diet for a little over six years. I was incredibly neurotic and militant about my diet. I wasn't even drinking tea at the time. Thank goodness I've relaxed a little bit and began adding cooked food to my diet again.

The main reason for my switching from an all-raw to a high-raw diet is that I feel more balanced when I reduce the amount of fats, nuts, and sugars I'm eating. Greens, beans, and grains are the staples of my current diet. With those three food groups, I feel better than I ever have. I feel grounded. When I see pictures of myself from when I was 100 percent raw, I notice that I looked too skinny, one-dimensional. And I remember feeling as if I was not in my body. It was hard to focus on everyday life or to create a successful business. I felt continually unstable when I was 100 percent raw. I also found that I was eating too much sugar and way too much fat at that time, influenced by the gourmet food dishes I was preparing.

I decided to reevaluate what the optimal diet for my body would be, what truly works for me. I have tried all sorts of cleanses, fasting, and a wide variety of raw foods, exploring what my body needs. At one time I was a fruitarian, then I went on the green diet, then I became gourmet raw, then simple raw. I went through many different phases, searching for what makes my body and mind feel the best. Living on an all-raw diet for six years had a major effect on my life in terms of influencing my thoughts around healing; I still think raw food is the most healing diet on the planet. If I were to get sick, I know it is best to go all raw, except that now I know to exclude dishes made with a lot of nuts and oils. If anybody I know gets sick, I will really encourage them to go all raw; but for everyday life, I believe incorporating some beans and grains into one's diet is beneficial. And in terms of being sustainable in the long run, it is almost unrealistic to live on a 100 percent raw diet. Most raw food diets are way too high in sugar and fat.

I've cut back on sugar and fat and eat whole food fats almost exclusively. For example, I don't eat oils or any other fractionated foods, and I eat very few nuts—on average, maybe one ounce or a small handful of nuts a day. Some days I'll have none, some days I'll have some, but nothing close to the ridiculous amount of nuts I used to consume as a 100 percent raw foodist. That seems very strange to me now. Considering that my diet was so calorie dense, it's hard to believe I wasn't gaining much weight.

Still, I believe there is a place for raw gourmet food in our lives. I think the raw gourmet style is highly influential and serves an amazing purpose in the culinary world. Raw gourmet food opens people's eyes to the greater possibilities of healthy eating; it helps people acknowledge vegetables as more than a side dish, and shows that healthy raw food can be just as comforting as any other meal, and is a great treat. I firmly believe that gourmet raw food should be acknowledged and honored on the same level as other types of cuisine. You eat French, you eat Italian, you eat raw food. Raw gourmet food is still my path and I still do the occasional event with that focus; I am just shifting my use of ingredients, that's all. I think gourmet raw food serves a major purpose in the mainstream and will continue to do so.

I first got into raw foods from a therapeutic point of view and then started to incorporate more gourmet raw dishes. But even while I was consuming gourmet raw, the foundation of my lifestyle was always cleansing, fasting, and incorporating lots of greens and green smoothies. Gourmet was such a small percentage of my diet; I never consistently ate just pâtés and pizzas and burritos. Salad has always been and continues to be the main staple of my diet. I still eat 80 percent raw. The other 20 percent is grains and beans rather than foods like nut pâtés.

When I travel around the world and teach or prepare food for people in other countries, I observe what other people eat on a daily basis and which foods are most beneficial for them. I came to the conclusion that the most beneficial diet is a whole-foods and plant-based diet, whether cooked or raw. High raw is preferable, but it depends on the season, the weather, and the availability of greens and fresh vegetables.

One thing that's been consistent in my diet is that I have stayed vegan since I became vegan. I can only speak for myself with that, but I do believe it is most beneficial for people to cut back on their intake of animal products, consuming them as little as possible and having plant-based dishes as the center of the meal. I've seen many people make this transition and get healthier, even healing some of their diseases.

Of course, people can make unhealthy choices on almost any kind of diet. Some kinds of cooked foods are more beneficial than some raw foods. When I joined Whole Foods Market I got my blood tested, which I had never done before. Several years ago I ate a lot of gourmet raw food but I hadn't eaten animal cholesterol in fifteen years. And my cholesterol was high! That blood test freaked me out. My triglycerides were off the chart. After that test, I went on a 100 percent whole food diet, free from all fractionated foods—no agave, no maple syrup, no coconut oil, no olive oil. I just focused on greens, beans, and grains. Within four months my cholesterol plummeted by almost 100 points and my triglycerides dropped. Now they are all below normal, which is perfect. On a typical raw food diet with some gourmet dishes, my blood results were showing me at high risk, even according to American standards, which is crazy and very humbling, because until I checked my blood I had always thought I was healthy. So I think it is very important for people to get their blood tested. Most people following a raw diet think that they're healthy because they're eating foods made from raw plants, nuts, and seeds, but a high-fat, high-sugar diet can raise your cholesterol.

Now I love beans. On average I eat about two cups per day, mixing it up with different kinds. I'll eat tofu maybe once a week; I don't eat a lot of soy. I use all sorts of legumes and ancient grains, getting creative, working with 100 percent whole foods, using nothing processed, not even coconut butter or agave. I still eat a few nuts and seeds and I eat plenty of avocados, olives, fresh coconuts, and other whole fats, but I don't eat oils, except on a rare occasion. When I prepare salads, I use avocado instead of oil. About 20 percent of my diet is cooked beans, greens, and grains, and I eat both raw and steamed greens. At home I don't cook with oil, at work I don't cook with oil anymore, and my cholesterol has remained low. I appreciate this totally new path of health that I am on now. It aligns with me and with the science and research, and it feels right.

I am happy that with this book we are giving people healthier options through delicious food. You can eat an omega-rich diet and still feel comforted. I think the information about oil and nuts is probably going to be the most controversial part of this book, which is exciting to me. It is going to be pretty shocking for our readers that all three of us well-known raw foodists have written a book that includes some cooked food. But I think people need to hear about what we've discovered through our personal experiences. With all of our recipes and articles and books over the years, our followers can see that we are on a journey just like everybody else, trying to find the healthiest diets for our bodies and passing that information on.

It's important to share this with people so they don't have to repeat our mistakes. People need to know that just because something is derived from a plant food doesn't mean that it is healthy. They need this knowledge so they don't stray down the wrong path of high fat and high sugar. I am glad to help with the paradigm shift. It has nothing to do with cooked this and raw that; at the end of the day, it's fractionated food that's the problem. It's food that is not real; it's not whole, not intact. The body can't recognize it. All oils contain 120–140 calories per tablespoon. When I was all raw, I was dumping four or five tablespoons of oil on my salad, and that was not healthy. Same thing with eating a pound or two of nuts per day. So I hope this book will shift people's minds and create controversy, which is fantastic.

I invite all my readers to assess what they are eating. Whole foods are real foods. Look into the program at Whole Foods Market called "Health Starts Here." I'm the coordinator of this global education program in the stores to guide customers to the healthiest options that Whole Foods sells. We've been trying to communicate through educational materials and programs. Look for the "Health Starts Here" logo at your local Whole Foods, or go to www.wholefoodsmarket.com. For more information you can also visit my website, www.rawchef.com.

PART TWO

Recipes

APPETIZERS, ANTIPASTI, AND FINGER FOODS

WALNUT FALAFEL WITH MINT TABOULI AND HEMP TZATZIKI

3 cups walnuts, soaked in water for at least a couple hours

3 dates, pitted and soaked for 2 hours

3/4 cup sesame seeds, finely ground

1/2 cup parsley, minced

1/2 cup cilantro, minced

1/2 tablespoon garlic, minced

3 tablespoons fresh oregano, minced

2 tablespoons lemon juice

1/4 teaspoon black pepper

2 teaspoons sea salt

In a Champion juicer or other juicer with a solid plate, blend the walnuts and dates. Mix in the remaining ingredients by hand. When thoroughly combined, form the mixture into small, half-dollar-size thumbprints and dehydrate for 4–6 hours or bake at 200° for 40 minutes. Serve with Fresh Mint Tabouli and Hemp Tzatziki (see below).

Fresh Mint Tabouli

1 cup tomatoes, diced

1/2 cup cucumber, diced

3 cups parsley, coarsely minced

1/2 cup parsnip, pulsed to approximately rice consistency

3 cloves garlic, minced

3 tablespoons mint chiffonade (To chiffonade, stack the leaves one on top of the other and roll tightly into a cylinder. Slice the cylinders of leaves crosswise into thin strips.)

3 tablespoons lemon juice

2 tablespoons lemon zest
3 tablespoons flaxseed oil
½ tablespoon sea salt

In a bowl, combine all the ingredients together. Let sit for the flavors to combine, ideally for 1 hour before serving.

Hemp Tzatziki

1 cup shelled hempseeds
3 tablespoons lemon juice
2 tablespoons hemp oil
½ teaspoon sea salt
2 cloves garlic
3 tablespoons water
2 tablespoons dill
1 tablespoon chives, minced
1 cup cucumber, seeded and diced

In a high-speed blender, blend the hempseeds, lemon juice, hemp oil, sea salt, garlic, and water until smooth. Stir in the dill, chives, and cucumber prior to serving.

∾ Chad

HEMP CROSTINI

3 ripe pears or sweet apples, peeled and chopped

1½ tablespoons walnut butter or hemp butter

3 tablespoons shelled hempseeds

2 tablespoons date paste or maple syrup

1 teaspoon sea salt

2 tablespoons onion powder

1 tablespoon onion flakes

2 tablespoons caraway seeds (preferably lightly toasted)

1 cup coarse flax meal

½ cup mix of dried coconut flour and almond flour

In a food processor, process the apple or pear, nut butter, and spices until a smooth consistency is reached. Pour in a tablespoon at a time of the flax meal and coconut/almond flour while processing until the mixture forms a ball. When you can roll the mixture into a ball by hand without it sticking, no more flour is needed. Form the ball into a small baguette and thinly slice it. Place the pieces of hemp bread on a dehydrator screen and dehydrate at 110° for 1–3 hours, or to desired texture. The bread will keep in the refrigerator for 1 week, or if dehydrated completely over 8 hours, it will keep for a month.

Note: Coconut flour is made by grinding dried, shredded coconut in a high-speed blender for 10–20 seconds and then straining it through a fine strainer or flour sieve. Coconut flour adds a subtle sweetness to the bread. Almond flour is made by dehydrating the pulp left over from making almond milk. Once dried, use a high-speed blender to grind until smooth.

~ *Chad*

CHEEZE WHIP

2 cups hempseeds or walnuts

1 clove garlic

1–2 tablespoons lemon juice

1 1/2 tablespoons mellow white miso paste

1/4 cup water or more to blend

1–3 teaspoons onion powder

2 tablespoons nutritional yeast flakes

1 carrot or 1 red bell pepper, chopped

If you are using walnuts, soak them for 12 hours and rinse well. Blend all the ingredients together until smooth and creamy. You may need to add more water to get the mixture smooth. For best distribution, place your Cheeze Whip in a quart-size storage bag and cut a small hole in one corner. Remove all the air and seal the top, then squeeze the mixture out the corner onto crackers or veggies.   ■ SERVES 4

Elaina

VALYA'S SALSA

RAW

4 large tomatoes, chopped
1/2 bunch cilantro, chopped
1 red bell pepper, finely chopped
1/2 bunch green onions, chopped
1 jalapeño pepper, diced
1/2 teaspoon salt
Juice of 1/2 lemon

Mix all ingredients and serve on crackers or veggies.

∾ *Valya*

MERLOT PICKLED ONIONS

RAW

2 red onions, peeled and sliced paper-thin on a mandoline

1/2 cup red wine or merlot vinegar

3 tablespoons agave

1 tablespoon flaxseed oil

Pinch of sea salt

Toss all the ingredients together well and gently knead. Set the mixture aside to pickle for at least a few hours, or overnight. Store in a jar and chill.

∾ *Chad*

MARINATED BABY VEGETABLES, FRESH CITRUS OLIVES, PICKLED GARLIC AND SWEET PEPPERS

Marinated Baby Vegetables

RAW

Baby whole carrots
Baby zucchini or baby pattypan squash
Baby beets, peeled and quartered

If baby vegetables are not available, simply substitute your choice of vegetables, sliced to the desired size.

Italian Marinade

$1/2$ cup flaxseed oil
$3/4$ cup apple cider vinegar
$1/2$ cup lemon juice
$1/4$ cup maple syrup
6 cloves garlic, finely minced
2 small shallots, finely minced
2 tablespoons fresh oregano, chopped
$1 1/2$ tablespoons fresh thyme, minced
1 red jalapeño or serrano chile, seeded and finely minced (optional)
$1 1/2$ tablespoons fine sea salt
$1/2$ tablespoon cracked black pepper

Whisk all the ingredients together well. Place the desired vegetables in a large sealable container and pour the marinade over them. Seal the container and place in the refrigerator overnight to marinate. Once marinated, strain and serve. You can use any leftover marinade as a salad dressing.

Fresh Citrus Olives

2 cups whole large green Sicilian olives
1 tablespoon finely grated (with microplane) orange zest
2 cloves garlic, finely minced
2 tablespoons oregano leaves, coarsely chopped
1/2 tablespoon dried chile flakes
Juice of 1/2 lemon

In a small bowl, toss all the ingredients together. Serve with antipasti. These are best if marinated overnight. The olives will keep for more than 2 weeks in the refrigerator.

Pickled Garlic and Sweet Peppers

2 red peppers, cored and sliced into 1/4-inch julienne or cubes
2 yellow peppers, cored and sliced into 1/4-inch cubes or julienned
Small handful of garlic cloves, coarsely chopped
1 1/2 tablespoons mixed peppercorns
4 bay leaves, dried or fresh
1 dried chile pepper
2 sprigs fresh oregano
1 tablespoon dill seed
1 tablespoon fine sea salt
3 cups apple cider vinegar
1 cup water

Set aside the sliced peppers and coarsely chopped garlic. In a quart-size mason jar, combine all the spices and herbs, except for the sea salt, and pack in the peppers and garlic. Top the peppers with the sea salt. Continue to pour in the apple cider vinegar until the jar is 2/3 full. Fill the remaining space in the jar with water. Tightly close the lid. Shake and leave in a dark place to pickle for at least 48 hours. This dish is best if left for 1 week to pickle, and will keep in the refrigerator for 1 month after pickling.

~ *Chad*

AVOCADO NORI ROLLS

Nori rolls make a great take-along meal. Avocado is a whole-raw fat that helps keep skin and hair soft and rids the body of toxic stored fats. Nori, the seaweed highest in protein content (48 percent), is very easily digested and extremely high in minerals.

Sushi

RAW

2 sheets of raw or toasted sushi nori

1 large romaine leaf, cut in half down the length of the spine

1 avocado, peeled and sliced

$1/2$ red, yellow, or orange bell pepper, julienned

$1/2$ cucumber, peeled, seeded, and julienned

$1/2$ cup raw sauerkraut

$1/2$ carrot, beet, or zucchini, shredded

1 cup alfalfa or favorite green sprouts (sunflower, buckwheat, etc.)

1 small bowl of water for sealing the roll

Spicy Miso Paste

4 tablespoons unpasteurized, mellow white miso

1 tablespoon sesame oil

$1/4$ teaspoon cayenne or to taste

Stir Spicy Miso Paste ingedients together with a fork.

Place a sheet of nori on a sushi rolling mat or washcloth, lining it up with the end of the sushi rolling mat closest to you. Place the romaine leaf on the edge of the nori, with the spine closest to you. Spread 1–2 tablespoons of Spicy Miso Paste on the romaine. Line the leaf with the ingredients in the order listed above, placing sprouts on last. Roll the nori sheet away from you, tucking the ingredients in with your fingers as you go. Seal the roll with water or Spicy Miso Paste and slice it into 6 rounds. ■ YIELDS 12 NORI ROLLS

∾ *Elaina*

SALADS

CAESAR SALAD

1 head of romaine, chopped
1 cucumber, peeled and cubed
1 tomato, chopped
4 scallions, thinly sliced
15 black olives, pitted

Dressing

$1/2$ cup flaxseed or hempseed oil
2 tablespoons lemon juice
$1/4$–$1/2$ cup water (start with $1/4$ cup and add more as needed)
2 large dates or 1 tablespoon Erythritol sugar-free sweetener
1 tablespoon mellow white miso paste
3 medium cloves garlic, crushed
$1 1/2$ teaspoons Dijon mustard
2 teaspoons dulse flakes
$1/4$ teaspoon sea salt

Blend all the ingredients together in a blender or mix by hand, whisking everything until well blended. Store in a glass jar in the refrigerator for up to 2 weeks. Toss together with salad.

Note: Try freeze-dried peas as croutons ... amazing!

∾ *Elaina*

PURPLE SALAD

RAW

1/4 head red cabbage, thinly sliced
1 grated carrot
1 grated Fuji apple
4 stalks of celery, chopped
1 pint blueberries
1 avocado, mashed
Juice of 1 lemon
1 tablespoon flaxseed, ground
1 tablespoon dulse flakes

Combine all the ingredients except the dulse flakes and flax-seed in a large bowl. Sprinkle the dulse flakes and freshly ground flaxseed on top and serve.　■ SERVES 2

∽ *Victoria*

TRIO OF CABBAGES WITH HEMP, AVOCADO, AND CILANTRO

RAW

2 cups finely shredded Napa cabbage

2 cups finely shredded red cabbage

2 cups finely shredded savoy or green cabbage

$1/4$ cup diced red and yellow bell peppers

3 tablespoons hemp oil

3 tablespoons lemon juice

3 tablespoons diced green onion

3 tablespoons cilantro leaves

1 teaspoon sea salt

2 avocados, diced

$1/4$ cup hulled hempseeds (lightly toasted preferred)

In a mixing bowl, toss all the ingredients except the hempseeds and the avocado together. As you mix, squeeze with your hands in order to wilt the cabbage. Gently mix the avocado into the salad and garnish with hempseeds. Serve immediately. As a variation, add fresh chopped herbs or your choice of diced vegetables. This dish is also delicious if kale, chard, or spinach is substituted for the cabbage. Note: Toss right before serving to retain crispness. ■ SERVES 4–6

∽ *Chad*

FENNEL, APPLE, AND ARUGULA WITH SUNFLOWER SPROUTS AND MANDARIN VINAIGRETTE

RAW

2–3 cups fennel bulbs, sliced paper-thin, preferably using a
    mandoline
1 cup fresh sunflower sprouts
1 cup baby arugula
Drizzle of Mandarin Vinaigrette (see p. 70)
2 pears or apples, sliced paper-thin, preferably using a
    mandoline
½ cup lightly dry-toasted pistachio meats
Merlot Pickled Onions (see p. 45)

In a small bowl, gently toss the shaved fennel, sunflower sprouts, and arugula with the Mandarin Vinaigrette. Prior to serving, garnish salad with a few slices of shaved pear or apple, toasted pistachios, and a scattering of pickled onions.

■ SERVES 4–6

∾ Chad

MARINATED CHARD AND KALE SALAD

A tender and delicious salad that has won the hearts of many doubters. If you've been reluctant to try raw kale, this is a good time to try it. It tastes better than you can imagine, and it's loaded with calcium, too!

Salad

RAW

1 bunch fresh kale (dinosaur, curly green, purple,
   or flat-leaf purple)
1 bunch Swiss chard (green-, yellow-, or red-stemmed)
1 medium red onion, sliced very thin
2 cloves garlic, crushed (optional)
2 medium avocados, cubed
1 medium zucchini or summer squash, julienned,
   or 10 shiitake mushrooms, thinly sliced
Dash of dried jalapeño or cayenne pepper

Marinade

$^3/_4$ cup flaxseed oil
$^1/_2$ cup lemon juice
1 teaspoon sea salt

Remove the stems of the kale and chard and tear the leaves into bite-size pieces. Pour the marinade over the leaves and mix together, squeezing the leaves well with your hands to help them become soft and tender. Add the rest of the salad ingredients and mix them together well, then allow the salad to marinate for another hour or more.

Note: The longer you allow the greens to marinate, the more tender they become. If you wish to prepare this salad in advance, it will keep for up to 5 days well sealed in your refrigerator; just don't add the avocados until serving time. For a creamy dressing, place the marinade ingredients in the blender with one of the avocados and blend. For variety, add a chunk of ginger to the blender.   ■ SERVES 4

∽ *Elaina*

ARUGULA SALAD

1 bunch fresh arugula
1/2 cup pitted olives
1/2 cup sliced pickles
1/2 cup fresh salsa (from the store or homemade)
1 pack frozen peas

Wash the arugula in a large bowl of water so that any particles of dirt sink to the bottom of the bowl and do not end up in your salad. Chop the arugula and place it in a salad bowl. Add the olives, pickles, and salsa. Place the frozen peas in a pan and fill it with water. Bring the peas to a boil, then immediately drain the water and mix the peas in with the rest of the ingredients.

■ SERVES 3

∿ *Valya*

FIELD GREENS WITH CARAMELIZED SHALLOTS, CANDIED WALNUTS, AND RASPBERRY VINAIGRETTE

RAW

5 cups mixed field greens

¼ cup chopped mixed herbs of your choice, such as parsley, dill, or basil

3 ounces (or desired amount) Raspberry Vinaigrette

3 tablespoons Caramelized Shallots

Small handful of Candied Walnuts (optional)

In a bowl, thoroughly mix all the ingredients except the candied walnuts together. Sprinkle the walnuts to garnish, and serve.

Raspberry Vinaigrette

1 cup raspberries

¼ cup apple cider vinegar

3 tablespoons flaxseed oil

2 cloves garlic

2 tablespoons ginger

1 tablespoon orange zest

1 teaspoon sea salt

2 tablespoons honey or maple syrup

In a high-speed blender, blend all the ingredients together well. The dressing will keep up to a week in the refrigerator.

Caramelized Shallots

1 cup shallots or red onions, sliced paper-thin with a mandoline

3 cloves garlic, minced

3 tablespoons flaxseed oil

3 tablespoons Nama Shoyu soy sauce

3 tablespoons date paste (pitted dates blended with water
    until a honey consistency is achieved)

Mix all the ingredients well in a bowl, coating the onions thoroughly with the marinade. Let sit for at least an hour. For best results, allow the mixture to marinate overnight. Strain off the excess liquid, spread the onions on a non-sticky sheet, and dehydrate for 1 hour until warm. Serve sprinkled on salads.

Candied Walnuts (or any nut/seed substitute)

2 cups walnuts, soaked in water for at least a couple hours

1/2 cup maple sugar

3 tablespoons orange zest

Pinch of cayenne

1/2 teaspoon sea salt

Toss all the ingredients together well and dehydrate for 12 hours or until crisp. Break into pieces and freeze to retain crispness.   ■ SERVES 4–6

∾ *Chad*

BEET SALAD

Grate the following vegetables:

RAW

1 large beet
1 large carrot
1 large cucumber
1 large Fuji apple

Add the following:

Juice of 1 lemon
1/2 small Hass avocado, mashed
1 cup spinach, thinly sliced
2 sprigs basil, chopped

Sprinkle the salad with 2–3 tablespoons sunflower seeds, soaked overnight. ■ SERVES 2

〰 *Victoria*

SWEET POTATO WEIGHT-LOSS SALAD

1 sweet potato, steamed

2 cups finely chopped celery

5 cherry tomatoes, quartered

$1/4$ teaspoon salt

2 cloves fresh garlic, chopped

$1/4$ teaspoon cayenne pepper

Use a fork to mash the sweet potato. Add the remaining ingredients, mix together, and serve. ■ SERVES 2

∾ *Valya*

SPROUT SALAD

2 cups sunflower sprouts

2 cups buckwheat sprouts

2 cups microgreens

2 green onions, chopped

$1/4$ teaspoon salt

1 teaspoon flaxseed oil

3 tablespoons nutritional yeast

Mix ingredients thoroughly in a large bowl.   ■ SERVES 2

~ *Valya*

A RIGHTEOUS SALAD

5 cups chopped baby greens

1 carrot, grated

1 tomato, chopped

4 radishes, sliced

1 cucumber, chopped

3 green onions, chopped

$1/2$ bunch fresh dill, chopped

$1/4$ teaspoon salt

4 tablespoons nutritional yeast

3 tablespoons salsa

$1/2$ cup pitted olives

Mix all the ingredients together in a large bowl and serve.

■ SERVES 3

∿ *Valya*

BELL PEPPER SALAD

4 red bell peppers, chopped

2 tablespoons nutritional yeast

$^1/_4$ teaspoon salt

$^1/_4$ bunch cilantro, chopped

2 green onions, chopped

1 teaspoon flaxseed oil (optional)

Mix all the ingredients together in a large bowl and serve.

■ SERVES 2

~ *Valya*

QUINOA SALAD

1 cup cooked quinoa

1 package frozen organic corn, brought to a boil and then
   drained

1 steamed zucchini, sliced

1 carrot, grated

1/2 bunch cilantro, chopped

1/4 bunch basil, chopped

1 medium tomato, chopped

2 cloves fresh garlic, minced

2 green onions, chopped

1/2 teaspoon salt

2 tablespoons nutritional yeast

Mix all the ingredients together in a large bowl and serve.

SERVES 3

∽ *Valya*

NOODLE SALAD WITH SWEET MISO-GINGER DRESSING

Dressing

RAW

½ cup flaxseed or hempseed oil

1 teaspoon toasted sesame oil (optional)

1 clove garlic

1 tablespoon grated fresh ginger

1 tablespoon apple cider vinegar or 2 tablespoons lemon juice

¼ cup raw honey or maple syrup (or sugar-free alternative: Erythritol)

2 tablespoons mellow white miso

2 teaspoons wheat-free tamari

Dash cayenne

¼ cup water

Salad

3 stalks broccoli, peeled and spiralized

2 large carrots, peeled and spiralized

2 zucchini or 1 English cucumber, spiralized

Place the dressing ingredients in a blender and process until smooth. Place the spiralized vegetables in a medium bowl. Just before serving, add the dressing to the vegetables and toss to combine. Serve immediately.　■ SERVES 4

~ *Elaina*

DRESSINGS

MANDARIN VINAIGRETTE

$^1/_2$ cup muscatel vinegar or white wine vinegar

$^1/_4$ cup flaxseed oil

2 tablespoons maple syrup

3 mandarin segments, diced

2 tablespoons finely chopped chives

2 tablespoons finely chopped mint

2 tablespoons orange zest

$^1/_4$ teaspoon ground black pepper

Whisk all ingredients together well.

∼Chad

FRESH VEGAN MAYO

1½ cups hempseeds

¾–1 cup water

1 teaspoon mustard

1 teaspoon sea salt

6 tablespoons lemon juice
   or 3 tablespoons apple cider vinegar

2 tablespoons raw honey or other sweetener

1½ cups Irish Moss Paste

Dash of cayenne pepper

1 clove garlic, crushed (optional)

1 teaspoon Italian seasoning or Bragg seasoning mix
   (optional)

1½ cups hemp, flax, or walnut oil

Place all the ingredients except the oil in a blender and blend until creamy. Then add the oil and blend again until well incorporated. Store in a glass jar. Will keep in the refrigerator for up to 2 weeks. ■ **YIELDS 6 CUPS**

IRISH MOSS PASTE

Irish moss is a health-promoting seaweed that can be used as a fat-free substitute for oil (try replacing ½ the oil in a recipe with this). It is a great thickener for desserts such as pies and cakes, and for shakes, too. You will see it used in this book in brownies, cookies, and pies. Try adding a tablespoon in your nut or seed milk to make it richer.

RAW

1 cup soaked Irish moss (about ½ cup before soaking)

½ cup purified water

Begin by rinsing the moss very well in water. Cover the moss in water in a large jar or bowl and let soak on the counter for 3 hours or overnight, rinsing well after soaking. The moss will get clearer and bigger the longer it is soaked. Rinse very well before using to remove the sea salt and dirt. Blend the purified water and moss on high speed until smooth. The paste will last in a glass jar in the refrigerator for up to 10 days. You may store the unblended, soaked moss out of water in an airtight container for 2 weeks or more. Moss doubles to triples in size once soaked.

∽*Elaina*

TOMATO-DILL DRESSING

1 cup chopped tomato

¼ cup hempseeds or olive oil

1 clove garlic

2 teaspoons lemon juice

⅓ teaspoon sea salt

¼ teaspoon thyme

1 tablespoon dried or 5 tablespoons fresh chopped dill weed

Blend until smooth.   ■ YIELDS 2 CUPS

∾ Elaina

RANCH DRESSING

1 cup hempseeds or walnuts

4 teaspoons lemon juice or 2$\frac{1}{2}$ teaspoons raw apple cider vinegar

1 teaspoon sea salt

1 teaspoon onion powder

1 teaspoon garlic powder

$\frac{3}{4}$ cup water

Blend until smooth before adding:

1 teaspoon dried dill weed

2 teaspoons Italian seasoning

■ YIELDS 2 CUPS

~ *Elaina*

RED BELL PEPPER DRESSING

RAW

1 large red bell pepper

1/2 cup chopped carrot

1 tablespoon grated or 1/2-inch piece ginger

1 clove garlic

5 small dates (for a low-sugar version, skip this step
   or add a couple drops of stevia)

Juice of 1 lemon or 2 teaspoons raw apple cider vinegar

1 teaspoon Celtic sea salt or 1 tablespoon tamari

1/2 cup flaxseed or hempseed oil

1/4 teaspoon kelp powder (optional)

Place all the ingredients in a blender and blend until smooth.
You may need to add a small amount of water. ■ YIELDS 2 CUPS

∽ Elaina

SOUPS

SPICY GREEN SOUP

3 cups stinging nettles (to avoid stinging during preparation,
   use gloves or a plastic bag)

1 cup mizuna

3 stalks celery, chopped

1 bunch cilantro

2 cups mustard greens

2 red bell peppers, chopped

1 avocado, peeled and seeded

Juice of 2 lemons

$\frac{1}{2}$ jalapeño pepper

4 cups water

Thoroughly blend all the ingredients in a blender. Serve with
dulse or other sea vegetables. ■ SERVES 3

Victoria

BUTTERNUT SQUASH SOUP

1 medium yellow onion, peeled and chopped

2 cloves garlic, chopped

2 teaspoons coconut oil

4 stalks celery, chopped

6 cups water (more or less)

1 medium butternut squash, peeled and chopped

1 head broccoli with peeled stem, chopped

1 red bell pepper, chopped (optional)

1–2 teaspoons curry powder or cumin powder

2–4 teaspoons Himalayan salt or to taste

Black pepper to taste

Cayenne to taste

10 large basil leaves

½ bunch cilantro

Sauté the onion and garlic in a large pot with the coconut oil. Add the celery and continue to sauté until the celery starts to soften. Add the water, butternut squash, and the remainder of the vegetables and spices, except for the fresh basil and cilantro. Let simmer for 10–15 minutes, then test the squash for softness. If it is soft enough to bite through, the soup is done. Adjust seasonings to taste. Remove ½–⅔ of the soup and blend it with the basil and cilantro until smooth. Add the blended mixture back to the pot with the unblended portion. Stir and serve.

∽ *Elaina*

WILD WEEDS SOUP

RAW

2 cups lambsquarters

1 cup mustard greens

1 cup purslane

1 avocado, peeled and seeded

Juice of 3 lemons

1 apple, chopped

4 cups water

1 tablespoon dulse flakes

Thoroughly blend all the ingredients except the dulse flakes in a blender. Serve sprinkled with dulse flakes. ■ SERVES 4

∾ *Victoria*

SIMPLY DELICIOUS PEA SOUP

1 bag frozen peas, defrosted
1½ cups hot water
1–2 teaspoons onion powder
1 teaspoon sea salt or to taste
2 teaspoons chia seeds or Jhempseeds
2 teaspoons flaxseed oil (optional)

Blend on high in a blender until smooth and serve immediately.

■ SERVES 4–6

∿ *Elaina*

ITALIAN SOUP

3 cups spinach

3 stalks celery, chopped

1 sprig basil

1 sprig thyme

1 red bell pepper, chopped

1 large avocado, peeled and seeded

1 cucumber, chopped

1 jalapeño pepper, chopped

Juice of 1 lime

2 cups water

1 tablespoon dulse flakes

Thoroughly blend all the ingredients except the dulse flakes together in a blender. Serve sprinkled with dulse flakes.

◾ SERVES 3

∾ *Victoria*

ROSEMARY RAIN SOUP

RAW

3 sprigs rosemary

2 stalks celery, chopped

1/2 bunch escarole

2 ripe tomatoes, cut in large pieces

1 cucumber, chopped

Juice of 3 limes

1 large avocado, peeled and seeded

3 cups water

1 tablespoon dulse flakes

Thoroughly blend all the ingredients except the dulse flakes together in a blender. Serve sprinkled with dulse flakes.

■ SERVES 4

∽ *Victoria*

CREAMY CILANTRO SOUP

Cilantro is a wonderfully fragrant herb that is high in chlorophyll and has been said to pull heavy metals from the body. Enjoy it in this rich and satisfying energy soup.

1 zucchini, chopped
1 large bunch cilantro, stems removed (about 2 cups)
1 red, yellow, or orange bell pepper, chopped
1/2 apple, chopped
1 avocado, chopped, or 1/4 cup soaked chia seeds
1 tablespoon tamari or Bragg Liquid Aminos
1 teaspoon Celtic sea salt
1/8 teaspoon cayenne
1/2 teaspoon cumin (optional)
1 teaspoon onion powder (optional)

Blend all the ingredients until smooth. Eat the soup immediately or store in a glass jar in the refrigerator for 1 day maximum.

Optional toppings: Sprinkle with dulse flakes, diced bell pepper, fresh corn cut off the cob, sunflower greens, or chopped romaine (stir into the soup).

SOAKED CHIA SEEDS

4 tablespoons chia seeds
2 cups purified water

Place the seeds in a 2-cup jar and pour the water over the seeds. Shake, cover, and refrigerate until needed, up to 1 week.

∿ *Elaina*

CELERY SOUP

RAW

6 stalks celery, chopped

4 ripe tomatoes, cut in large pieces

1/2 avocado, peeled and seeded

Juice of 2 lemons

4 cups water

1 cup alfalfa sprouts

2 tablespoons dulse flakes

Thoroughly blend all the ingredients except the sprouts and the dulse flakes in a blender. Serve with sprouts and sprinkled with dulse flakes.　　　　　■ SERVES 4

∾ *Victoria*

MUSHROOM-POTATO SOUP

1 1/2 cups potatoes, washed and diced

6 cups water

2 cups celery, diced

1 cup tomatoes, diced

1 hot pepper or 1 teaspoon ground cayenne pepper, or to taste

1 cup button mushrooms, diced

1/3 cup onion, finely chopped

1 cup diced parsley or basil, or any other herb

1 tablespoon miso

1 tablespoon dulse flakes

Place the potatoes in water in a stockpot. Bring to a boil, then cook over medium heat until the potatoes are tender, about 5–10 minutes. Add celery, tomatoes, pepper, mushrooms, and onion. Bring to a boil. Add the parsley and immediately remove the soup from heat. Stir in the miso and sprinkle with dulse flakes. ■ SERVES 6

∽ *Victoria*

VEGETABLE SOUP WITH LENTILS

1 cup dry lentils, rinsed

12 cups water

1 potato, peeled and diced

1 carrot, diced

2 cups celery, diced

1 cup tomatoes, diced

1 hot pepper or 1 teaspoon ground cayenne pepper, or to taste

1 bunch green onions, chopped

2 cups bok choy, chopped

1 bunch fresh cilantro, chopped

1 tablespoon miso

1 tablespoon flaxseed oil

1 tablespoon dulse flakes

Soak lentils overnight in 6 cups water. In the morning drain that water and rinse lentils well. Place them in a stockpot. Add 6 cups fresh water to the lentils and bring to a boil, stirring occasionally. Cover and simmer for 25–30 minutes or until the lentils are cooked. Add the potatoes and bring them to a boil, then cook over medium heat until they are tender, about 5–10 minutes. Add the carrot, celery, tomatoes, pepper, and onion, and again bring the soup to a boil. Add the bok choy and cilantro and immediately remove the soup from heat. Stir in miso. Serve with flaxseed oil and dulse flakes.   ■ SERVES 6

෴ *Victoria*

QUICK BORSCHT

COOKED

1 beet, scrubbed and diced

6 cups water

1 potato, peeled and diced

2 cups red cabbage, diced

2 cups celery, diced

2 cups Italian kale or collards, washed and chopped

1 hot pepper or 1 teaspoon ground cayenne pepper, or to taste

3 cloves garlic, peeled and diced

1 bunch fresh parsley, chopped

1 tablespoon miso

Juice of 1 medium lemon

1 tablespoon flaxseed oil

1 tablespoon dulse flakes

Place the beets in water and bring to a boil. Cover and simmer for 10 minutes. Add the potatoes and bring to a boil, then cook over medium heat until they are tender, about 5–10 minutes. Add the cabbage, celery, kale, and pepper, and again bring the soup to a boil. Add the garlic and parsley and immediately remove the borscht from heat. Stir in miso and lemon juice. Serve with flaxseed oil and dulse flakes. ■ SERVES 6

∾ *Victoria*

GARDEN MINESTRONE
WITH WILD RICE AND SAGE PESTO

½ cup sun-dried tomatoes, soaked for 2 hours

3 cloves garlic

2 cups water (preferably the tomato soak water)

3 cups tomatoes, chopped

½ cup parsley, chopped

⅓ cup basil, chopped

3 stalks celery, chopped

1 zucchini, chopped

1 tablespoon oregano, minced

1 apple, diced

1 tablespoon sea salt

¼ teaspoon cayenne

Dash of white pepper

2 cups wild rice, sprouted

1 cup diced portobello, marinated in 2 tablespoons of Nama
   Shoyu soy sauce or tamari for 1 hour or until soft (optional)

In a Vitamix blender with variable speeds or in a food processor, blend sun-dried tomatoes, garlic, and one cup of water until smooth. Add the remaining ingredients except the rice and mushrooms. Blend on low, not liquefying but leaving a slightly chunky consistency. Add the rice and blend on low for 10–15 seconds. Pour into a saucepan and stir in the marinated portobellos. Serve warm with Sage Pesto. ■ SERVES 4

WILD RICE SOFTENING
This method softens the rice and gives it a nutty flavor. Put the wild rice in a jar with a sprouting lid to make the process

easier and the cleanup quicker. Soak the wild rice in filtered water for 10–12 hours, at room temperature. Strain the rice and continue to rinse twice a day for 2–3 days. To ensure the rice is well rinsed, make sure the water is clear after rinsing. The rice is good after a day of rinsing, but will soften more if soaked for an additional couple days. You may use this rice in salads, stir-fries, and soups.

Sage Pesto

1 cup fresh basil, chopped
1/4 cup leeks, chopped
2 tablespoons fresh sage, chopped
3 tablespoons fresh oregano, chopped
1/2 cup walnuts or hempseeds
2 cloves garlic, chopped
1/2 tablespoon sea salt
3 tablespoons nutritional yeast
Cracked or coarsely ground pepper to taste
3 tablespoons flaxseed oil or olive oil

In a food processor, add all the ingredients except the oil. Blend together while slowly adding the oil to the mixture. Do not blend until completely smooth as this should be a "rustic" pesto that has some texture. Add a dollop to the minestrone soup before serving.

∾ Chad

MISO BROTH WITH COCONUT SOBA

4 cups coconut water

$1/4$ cup dark barley miso

2 tablespoons tamari or Nama Shoyu soy sauce

1 tablespoon sesame oil

2 cloves garlic

$1 1/2$ tablespoons ginger, chopped

1 tablespoon lemongrass, chopped (optional)

$1/3$ cup coconut meat, julienned thin to noodle size (if not available, use zucchini, peeled and julienned or spiralized into "noodles")

1 carrot, julienned paper-thin

$1/4$ cup snow peas, julienned paper-thin

$1/4$ cup red bell pepper, diced

2 tablespoons spring onion, diced

2 tablespoons toasted sesame seeds

In a high-speed blender, blend the coconut water, miso, tamari, sesame oil, garlic, ginger, and lemongrass until liquefied, then slowly pour the mixture through a fine-mesh strainer. Combine with the coconut meat, carrot, snow peas, and red bell pepper in a small soup pot and heat. Serve this soup warm, ensuring the vegetables remain crisp. Garnish with diced spring onion and toasted sesame seeds. ■ SERVES 4–6

~ *Chad*

YELLOW SPLIT PEA SOUP
WITH SMOKED DULSE AND KALE

COOKED

3 tablespoons olive oil

1 white onion, diced

4 cloves garlic, chopped

1 1/2 cups yellow split peas

6 cups low- or no-sodium vegetable stock

1/2 cup whole-leaf dulse seaweed (preferably applewood-smoked), ripped into 1-inch pieces

2 tablespoons fresh thyme, minced

3 tablespoons parsley, chopped

3 tablespoons fresh lemon juice

1/2 tablespoon sea salt (or more to taste)

1/2 cup nutritional yeast

1 teaspoon fresh cracked black pepper

2 cups kale of your choice, shredded

Add the oil to a soup pot over medium heat. When the oil is hot, toss in the onions, cooking them until translucent, then add the garlic. Add the split peas and 5 cups vegetable stock (reserve the other cup for later, if needed once the peas are cooked). Bring to a simmer and allow to cook for 12–15 minutes. Add the dulse, thyme, parsley, lemon juice, sea salt, nutritional yeast, and pepper. Add the remaining cup of vegetable stock if needed to thin, and cook for an additional 5–8 minutes. Add the kale, remove the soup from heat, and put on the lid. Allow the kale to steam for 5–10 minutes from the heat of the soup. Stir and serve. Best served with your favorite seeded whole-grain bread. Garnish with fresh parsley and a lemon wedge. ■ **SERVES 4–6** (If not served as the entrée, there will be leftovers.)

∽ *Chad*

BREADS, CRACKERS, AND CHIPS

BROWN WALNUT BREAD

2¹/₄ cups packed walnut pulp (This is leftover pulp from
making nut milk. You can use any nut or seed pulp you have
on hand.)

³/₄ cup ground chia seeds or flaxseeds

¹/₃ cup carob or cacao powder (I prefer carob)

³/₄ teaspoon sea salt

2 tablespoons caraway seeds (more or less according to taste)

¹/₂ cup walnut oil

¹/₂ cup sauerkraut (add more for a more sour taste)

Mix the dry ingredients together with your hands first, then stir in the oil and sauerkraut and stir together until well combined. Roll out half of the batter and sandwich between two 14 x 14-inch non-sticky sheets. Use a rolling pin or olive oil bottle to flatten and even out the batter. Remove the top non-sticky sheet and use a pastry scraper to spread the dough out to the edges of the sheet and make it square. Score the bread into 16 squares (approximately 3 x 3-inch) per tray and then flip it onto a dehydrator tray with the screen in place. (The tray will have no non-sticky sheets on the top or bottom, just the screen and tray.) Dehydrate for about 4 hours at 110°. You will know the bread is ready when it is moist but not doughy. Store in a plastic bag or glass container in the refrigerator for 4–5 days or in the freezer for 2–4 weeks. This bread will not stay fresh long at room temperature since it is not dried completely, but it should keep overnight.   ■ YIELDS 24 PIECES

∾ *Elaina*

CILANTRO-WALNUT CRACKERS OR DIP

5 cups soaked walnuts (2^1/2 cups before soaking)
1 clove garlic, minced
1 tablespoon grated ginger
^{1}/4 cup packed cilantro leaves
2 stalks celery, chopped
1 green onion, chopped
1 teaspoon Celtic sea salt
Juice of 1 or 2 lemons (3–6 tablespoons juice)
1 cup flax or chia seeds, ground into meal

Purée everything except the flax or chia meal in a food processor until well puréed but not completely smooth. Stir in flax meal. Eat as a dip or make into crackers. For crackers: Spread the mixture evenly onto a dehydrator tray lined with a non-sticky sheet. Dehydrate at 105° for 8 hours. Flip the crackers over, remove the non-sticky sheet, and dehydrate for another 12 hours or until crunchy. Store the crackers in a glass jar after they have cooled.

～Elaina

OMEGA-3 BIRDSEED FLAX CRACKERS

RAW

1 cup black chia seeds

2 cups golden flaxseeds

2 cups brown flaxseeds

3 cups hempseeds

15 cups water

2$\frac{1}{2}$ teaspoons Himalayan salt

Rinse all the seeds well, then mix all the seeds together and soak in a large bowl of water. Stir the seeds again after about 1 hour of soaking. Do not try to rinse the seeds again once they have been soaked as you may rinse off the gelatinous properties. After 4–8 hours of soaking, hand mix in the Himalayan salt, stirring well. Spread 2$\frac{1}{2}$ cups batter onto a 14 x 14-inch non-sticky-sheet-lined dehydrator tray. Score into 25–36 crackers per tray using a metal pastry scraper (Bash N Chop) or a metal, offset spatula. Dehydrate for 2 hours at 140°. Turn the temperature down to 105° and continue to dehydrate for another 6 hours or so until the non-sticky sheet comes off easily. Flip the crackers over onto a screen that has no non-sticky sheet on it and remove the non-sticky sheet from the back of the crackers. Continue to dry until the crackers are crunchy (about 24–36 hours altogether). Store in an airtight glass container after they have cooled. These will keep for 3 months unrefrigerated or 6 months refrigerated or frozen.

∿ *Elaina*

CRUNCHY CHIA CRISPS

4 cups chia seeds

10 cups water

2 teaspoons sea salt

1 red bell pepper, chopped

1 zucchini, chopped

6 stalks celery, chopped

2 small tomatoes, chopped

2 teaspoons grated ginger

In a large bowl, pour the water over the chia seeds and stir well. After 15 minutes, stir again to be sure the seeds soak evenly. Let the seeds soak 4 hours or overnight at room temperature. The seeds will absorb all the water, so there is no need to rinse or drain them at this point. Purée the vegetables in a food processor, leaving them a little bit chunky. Add all the ingredients together into the bowl of soaked chia seeds and mix well with a large spoon. Using an offset metal spatula or scraper like the Bash N Chop tool, spread 3 cups batter onto dehydrator trays that have been lined with non-sticky sheets. Dehydrate for 8 hours, or until the crisps seem ready to flip, and remove the sheet. Continue to dehydrate until the crisps are crunchy and completely dry. Let cool for 5–10 minutes or until cooled completely. Store in an airtight container to preserve freshness and crispness.

Shelf life: Frozen or refrigerated: 6 months. Cool, dark cupboard: 3 months.

Variations: To vary the flavor, add a combination of your favorite herbs and spices in equal amounts. For a variety of colors and flavors, change the vegetables to cabbage, beets, carrots, etc.

For other variations, hand mix some or all of the following into the Crunchy Chia Crisps recipe:

2 teaspoons curry powder

2 teaspoons cumin powder

1/4 cup tomato powder

2 cloves garlic, crushed or minced

1 bunch cilantro, chopped

ᴄᴏ *Elaina*

KALE CHIPS

Kale chips are like potato chips with all of the crunch and flavor and none of the guilt! Try a head of curly kale with either of these variations.

RAW

1 large head curly kale

Tomato-Dill

1 cup tomato, chopped
$1/4$ cup hempseeds
1 clove garlic
2 teaspoons lemon juice
$3/4$ teaspoon sea salt
$1/4$ teaspoon thyme
1 tablespoon dried dill weed or 5 tablespoons fresh chopped
   dill weed

Ranch

1 cup hempseeds or walnuts
4 teaspoons lemon juice or $2^1/2$ teaspoons raw apple cider
   vinegar
1 teaspoon sea salt
1 teaspoon onion powder
1 teaspoon garlic powder
$1/2$ cup water

Blend Ranch ingredients until smooth before adding:

1 teaspoon dried dill weed
2 teaspoons Italian seasoning

Wash 1 large head of curly kale and dry well. Blend all the ingredients together (except kale) until smooth. Use the whole leaves and stems of the kale (or beet tops or collards), keeping the leaves as whole as possible. Toss the dressing together with the greens in a bowl and mix until the leaves are coated. Place on dehydrator trays that have been lined with non-sticky sheets and dehydrate for 4 or more hours at 105°. Remove the non-sticky sheets and continue drying about 3 more hours or until crisp. Let cool completely before storing in a glass jar for up to a month. (*Note:* Storing these chips in a ziplock bag will make them go stale within 12 hours!)

∽ *Elaina*

CHIPOTLE TOSTADAS

SOME COOKED

Organic sprouted corn tortillas

2 cups Fat-Free Chipotle Red Beans (see p. 115)

1 avocado, thinly sliced

2 small tomatoes, chopped

$1/4$ cup minced cilantro

$1/4$ cup salsa

4 leaves romaine lettuce, thinly sliced

Toast the tortillas in a toaster oven or bake at 250° for 15 minutes, or until golden and crispy. Start assembling your tostadas by placing a dollop of beans on a tortilla, then layer your ingredients, finishing with the lettuce. ■ SERVES 2

ᔕ *Elaina*

ENTRÉES

ZUCCHINI PASTA WITH ARUGULA-PESTO SAUCE

Pasta

RAW

4 zucchini, cut into fine noodles on a mandoline
  or spiral slicer

Sauce

½ cup walnuts
½ cup basil leaves, tightly packed
½ cup arugula leaves, tightly packed
1 teaspoon lemon juice
3–5 cloves garlic, minced
1 tablespoon mellow white miso paste
½ teaspoon sea salt
¼ cup flaxseed or hempseed oil
Pine nuts for sprinkling

Soak the walnuts 2–24 hours, then rinse well. Purée all sauce
ingredients in a food processor or blender until smooth. Toss
with the noodles and sprinkle with pine nuts.

Additional items you can mix in or top your pasta with:
chopped olives, soaked and chopped sun-dried tomatoes, fresh
chopped tomatoes, nutritional yeast, or dulse flakes.

■ SERVES 4

∾ Elaina

LENTILS IN HEAVEN

COOKED

2½ cups red lentils, soaked overnight
4 cups water

Bring the water to a boil in a stockpot and add the lentils. Stir right away to keep the lentils from sticking to the bottom of the pan. After 15 minutes add:

½ medium sweet potato, peeled and cubed
½ medium yam, peeled and cubed
1 medium potato, cubed
7 large cloves garlic, peeled
½ teaspoon cayenne pepper
½ teaspoon salt

Continue cooking for 10 more minutes at a low boil or until potatoes are done. Add 3 tablespoons lemon juice. Sprinkle with diced green onions and fresh dill. ■ SERVES 3

∽ *Valya*

FIRE-ROASTED TOMATO LENTIL CHILE WITH AVOCADO CRÈME AND BROWN RICE

2 tablespoons olive oil

1 large onion, diced

4 cloves garlic, minced

1 fresh jalapeño pepper, minced

1 cup green lentils

1 cup sweet potato, peeled and $1/2$-inch diced

3 celery stalks, sliced in half lengthwise then chopped

2 cups low-sodium vegetable stock

1 16-ounce can fire-roasted diced tomatoes with juice, no salt added

$1/2$ tablespoon smoked paprika

$1/2$ tablespoon cumin powder

3 tablespoons cilantro, chopped

2 tablespoons maple syrup

2 cups winter greens (kale, collards, Swiss chard, cabbage, mustard greens), torn into 1-inch pieces

Sea salt and freshly ground black pepper to taste

In a large pot on medium-high heat, add the oil and onions, stirring continuously until translucent. Add the garlic and fresh jalapeño peppers and continue to cook until the peppers are browned. Add the lentils, sweet potato, celery, and vegetable stock. Simmer for 10 minutes. Add the canned tomatoes, herbs, spices, and greens. Cover and simmer for 5–8 minutes. Remove from heat and allow to sit before serving so the flavors combine. Season to taste, adding sea salt and pepper if desired. Serve with a dollop of Avocado Crème and chopped green onions over brown rice.

Avocado Crème

3 avocados, peeled and seeded
3 cloves garlic
$1/4$ cup lime juice
$1/2$ cup hempseeds
3 tablespoons flaxseed oil
Sea salt

In a food processor, blend the ingredients until smooth, adding the flaxseed oil while blending to create a smooth crème. Serve chilled with Fire-Roasted Tomato Lentil Chile.

■ SERVES 6–8

∽ *Chad*

WILD MUSHROOM CROQUETTES
WITH RUSTIC PUTTANESCA

Croquettes

RAW

3 cups walnuts, soaked 10–12 hours

1 cup pine nuts

3 portobello mushroom caps, diced and marinated in 2
   tablespoons Nama Shoyu soy sauce and 2 tablespoons
   olive oil for 1 hour or until soft

3 celery stalks, diced

$1/4$ cup red onion, minced

$1/3$ cup cherry tomatoes, halved

1/3 cup small broccoli florets

$1^{1}/2$ tablespoons dried thyme

$1^{1}/2$ tablespoons dried sage

$1/3$ cup fresh basil leaves, torn into small pieces

3 tablespoons fresh oregano, minced

2 tablespoons lemon juice

1 tablespoon chile powder

$1/2$ tablespoon sea salt

Dash of cracked black pepper

Grind the nuts and set aside. Marinate the diced portobellos
and set them aside for 1 hour or until soft. Add the remaining ingredients to the nut mixture. When the diced portobellos
are soft, toss them into the mixture along with the marinade.
Stir everything together until thoroughly combined. On a nonsticky sheet, form into 4-inch patties and dehydrate at 110° for
4–6 hours.

Rustic Puttanesca

1/4 cup mixed olives (Kalamata, green, and black), pitted and
  coarsely chopped
3 tablespoons capers, rinsed
1/2 cup sun-dried tomatoes, rehydrated and julienned
3 tablespoons olive oil
2 tablespoons lemon zest
2 cloves garlic, minced
1 small red onion, finely diced
1 fresh red chile, minced
Sea salt and pepper to taste

In a bowl, combine the olives, capers, and sun-dried tomatoes
and mix them together thoroughly with the remaining ingredients. Serve over Wild Mushroom Croquettes. ■ SERVES 6

~ Chad

THAI BROCCOLI WITH ALMOND CHILE SAUCE AND ROOT RICE

Thai Broccoli

RAW

½ cup almond butter

1 tablespoon ginger, chopped

1½ tablespoons lemon juice

2 tablespoons sweetener (dates, raisins, or prunes)

2 cloves garlic

2 tablespoons tamari or Nama Shoyu soy sauce

1 serrano pepper, diced (optional)

⅓ cup water (or more if needed) to thin

3 cups broccoli florets, chopped

½ cup red and yellow bell peppers, diced

½ cup cilantro, chopped

1 cup Asian bean sprouts

In a high-speed blender, blend the almond butter, ginger, lemon juice, sweetener, garlic, tamari sauce, serrano pepper, and water until smooth. Add more water if needed for desired consistency. Toss the sauce in a large bowl with the chopped broccoli, peppers, cilantro, and bean sprouts. After the vegetables are well combined, dehydrate them on non-sticky sheets at 105° for 2–3 hours to soften. Serve over Root Rice. ■ SERVES 4

Root Rice: Parsnip and Sesame

6 cups parsnips, peeled

½ cup pine nuts

3 tablespoons flaxseed oil

1 tablespoon toasted sesame oil

1 tablespoon sea salt
1 teaspoon black pepper
3 tablespoons chives, minced
2 tablespoons black sesame seeds

In a food processor, pulse all the ingredients until minced to a white-rice consistency. Use this as a base or serve on a plate with the Thai Broccoli.   ■ YIELDS 7 CUPS

~ *Chad*

MARINATED VEGETABLE LASAGNA

Red Bell Marinara

2 cups sun-dried tomatoes covered in water for 2 or more
hours (save the water for a salad dressing or possibly to
thin the sauce)
2 large dates or 1 tablespoon Erythritol
2 cloves garlic
1/8 red onion, chopped
6 basil leaves
1 large bell pepper (or 1 medium tomato), chopped
1 teaspoon Himalayan salt
1/8 teaspoon oregano

Blend everything in a blender or purée in a food processor until smooth.

Ricotta

3 1/2 cups walnuts, soaked 24 hours
1/2 cup water (or more as needed)
2 cloves garlic, minced
1/4 cup light miso paste
2 tablespoons lemon juice
1 teaspoon Italian seasoning

Soak the walnuts for 24 hours, rinse very well, and drain. Purée all the ingredients in a food processor or blend until fluffy.

Vegetables

4 medium yellow or green zucchini, thinly sliced lengthwise on
a mandoline

2 large portobello mushrooms, chopped and marinated in
    tamari or lemon juice and salt for 1 hour or until soft
1 large bunch or 4 cups spinach, washed, dried, and pulsed
    in a food processor
2 cups arugula, washed, dried, and pulsed in a food processor
1 large red bell pepper and 1 large yellow bell pepper,
    julienned and chopped then dehydrated for 1 or more hours

Mix pulsed spinach with pulsed arugula in a separate bowl.

Layering

Place enough zucchini slices on the bottom of a square (9 x 9-inch) glass pan to cover it. Layer on ⅓ of the marinara sauce, then ⅓ of the ricotta, using your fingers or a pastry bag if necessary to spread evenly. Then, using your hands or a nut milk bag, squeeze all the liquid out of the mushrooms and layer half of them on the cheese (you can pulse them in a food processor to make a meaty texture if desired). Squeeze the liquid out of the pulsed spinach-arugula mixture using a nut milk bag, and layer half onto the mushrooms. Then add half of the bell peppers. Start again with the zucchini, sauce, ricotta, mushrooms, spinach-arugula, and peppers. Keep layering until you run out of ingredients or room in your pan, and finish with the cheese and finally the sauce, swirling it together so that when you dehydrate it, the dish looks like baked lasagna. You can also make your lasagna in a springform pan. Remove the side of the pan and it looks like a fancy vegetable terrine! If it's a sunny day, place the lasagna in the sun with a dehydrating screen on top for a couple hours; otherwise, warm it in the dehydrator on 125° for a couple hours.   ■ SERVES 8

෴ *Elaina*

STEAMED VEGGIES

3 cups green beans
4 baby bok choy, chopped
1 carrot, sliced
1/4 red cabbage, sliced
5 mushrooms, chopped
3 cups broccoli chunks

Steam all the veggies, adding the mushrooms and broccoli last.

Add the following seasonings:

2 tablespoons nutritional yeast
1/2 teaspoon salt
1/2 teaspoon coriander
1/2 teaspoon cayenne pepper
1/2 teaspoon onion powder

Mix and serve. ■ SERVES 6

∾ *Valya*

FAT-FREE CHIPOTLE RED BEANS

COOKED

2 cups red beans (about 3 cups after sprouting), soaked and
then sprouted to $1/4$-inch tails (see directions below)

5 cups water

2 cloves garlic, chopped

$1/4$ onion, chopped

1 piece kombu seaweed

2 teaspoons sea salt

2 dashes cayenne pepper

1 teaspoon cumin powder

2 chipotle chiles (optional)

1 tablespoon tomato powder

Soak the beans overnight, or for at least 6 hours. Sprout them
by straining in a colander or nut milk bag and rinsing them
every morning and evening for two days or until $1/4$-inch tails
form. In a medium pot, cook all the ingredients together for
1–2 hours or until the beans are soft. Serve whole or blend all
the ingredients together in a food processor to make a refried
bean texture. Enjoy on tostadas or wrapped in a romaine lettuce leaf. ■ SERVES 3

∾ *Elaina*

MAC 'N' CHEEZE

RAW

4 zucchini, peeled
1 teaspoon sea salt
1 batch of Cheeze Whip (see p. 43)

Using the large blade on a spiralizer (Paderno or Spirooli are a couple of different brand names for this tool), spiralize your zucchini into noodles, then cut them into 2-inch lengths with scissors. Toss with the salt and let sit about 5 minutes or until the zucchini begins to weep. Spin in a salad spinner until all the excess liquid is removed. Mix with the Cheeze Whip and enjoy. ■ SERVES 3

↝ *Elaina*

MARINATED TENDER BROCCOLI AND ZUCCHINI

Vegetables for Marinade

RAW

2 heads of broccoli
2 zucchini, sliced into thin half-moons or matchsticks
¼ red bell pepper, minced
5 very thin slices of red onion, quartered

Cut the broccoli into bite-size spears. Peel the fibrous pieces with a paring knife.

Marinade

½ cup filtered water
2 teaspoons sea salt
½ cup flaxseed oil
2 tablespoons fresh rosemary
2 tablespoons miso
4 cloves garlic
2 tablespoons onion powder
2 tablespoons lemon juice
1 tablespoon wheat-free tamari

Blend until smooth. Mix with the vegetables and let marinate for 5 or more hours. To speed up the process, place the vegetables into a quart-size glass jar and press them firmly down into the liquid. Dehydrate at 105° until they are tender. For the best flavor, serve the vegetables warmed in the dehydrator.

■ SERVES 6

∾ *Elaina*

DESSERTS

LOW-GLYCEMIC OMEGA-3 COFFEE "ICE CREAM"

4 cups hempseed or walnut milk (2$\frac{1}{2}$ cups nuts or seeds
blended with 4 cups water)

$\frac{3}{4}$ cup Irish Moss Paste (see pp. 71–72)

$\frac{1}{4}$ cup maple syrup

$\frac{3}{4}$ cup Erythritol, Lakanto, or Xylitol sweetener

10 drops coffee essence

10 drops vanilla essence

$\frac{1}{4}$ teaspoon salt

$\frac{1}{4}$ teaspoon liquid stevia

$\frac{1}{4}$ cup coconut oil

Make the milk by blending the water and nuts or seeds together, then strain the liquid through a nut milk bag. Put the nut pulp in the freezer for an alternate use. Mix the nut milk and remaining ingredients together and pour into an ice-cream maker.

I prefer the Cuisinart Ice Cream Maker with a freezable cylinder. Freeze the cylinder overnight for best results. Remove the cylinder from the freezer and assemble the machine with the spinning paddle in place. Turn the machine on, then pour the "Ice Cream" batter into the frozen cylinder. Let run for 20–30 minutes or until the mixture is frozen into a fairly hard ice "cream." For best results, don't run longer than 40 minutes or the mixture will begin to defrost. Serve immediately or store in the freezer.

Tip: ¾ cup of liquid serves one person so I like to save the liquid in the refrigerator and only make enough to eat at one time. This ice cream does not freeze well long-term. The ice-cream batter will last refrigerated for 5 days. ■ SERVES 10–12

෴ *Elaina*

VALYA'S SILLY-YUM SORBET

RAW

2 cups fresh orange juice

1 frozen banana

1 cup frozen strawberries

1 cup frozen cherries

4 tablespoons psyllium husk powder

Place all the ingredients in a high-speed blender. Using a tamper, blend thoroughly on low or medium speed. It is not necessary to blend this sorbet on maximum speed. Also, using a low or medium speed will be easier on your blender. Have glasses ready to pour the sorbet into as soon as it is done blending, as the psyllium is a thickener and will quickly firm up. ■ SERVES 3

∿ Valya

THE HAPPY COLON SORBET

RAW

2 cups fresh apple juice

1 frozen banana

1 cup frozen peaches

1 cup frozen blueberries

4 tablespoons psyllium husk powder

Place all the ingredients in a high-speed blender. Using a tamper, blend thoroughly on low or medium speed. It is not necessary to blend this sorbet on maximum speed. Also, using a low or medium speed will be easier on your blender. Have glasses ready to pour the sorbet into as soon as it is done blending, as the psyllium is a thickener and will quickly firm up. ■ SERVES 3

∾ Valya

PINK GRAPEFRUIT CREAM SORBET DECADENCE

2 pink grapefruit (1½ cups juice)

½ cup coconut palm sugar or yacón root syrup, or your
favorite healthy sweetener

2 teaspoons lemon or lime juice

¼ teaspoon sea salt

1 tablespoon ground chia seeds

1 teaspoon powdered soy lecithin

Wash the grapefruit well with water and dish soap. Using a zester or microplane, remove the zest from the peel of one grapefruit. Squeeze enough juice from the grapefruit to make 1½ cups juice. Strain the seeds out of the juice using a nut milk bag or sieve. Add all the ingredients together in a blender and blend well. Taste the mixture after blending. Since some grapefruits are sweeter than others, you may need to add additional sweetener in the form of a few drops of stevia. Freeze the grapefruit mixture in a 2- or 4-quart ice-cream freezer according to the manufacturer's directions. ■ **YIELDS 3 CUPS**

∾ *Elaina*

BLACK FOREST CAROB BROWNIES

4 cups soaked and dehydrated (optional) walnuts

³/₄ cup pitted dates

³/₄ cup carob powder or 1 cup raw cacao powder

2 teaspoons cherry or vanilla extract

¹/₂ cup coarsely chopped dried walnuts

¹/₂ cup coarsely chopped dried cherries

Soak the walnuts for 8–12 hours. Rinse them well and dry them with a towel. Dehydrate the walnuts in a food dehydrator at 105° for 12 hours. (This is an optional step that will give the brownies a more cakelike texture.) Purée the nuts in a food processor until they become a flour. Add the dates and continue to purée until the mixture is well combined. Add the carob powder and extract, and purée again. Mix in the chopped nuts and cherries by hand. With very firm pressure, press the mixture into a brownie pan. Refrigerate for an hour, then slice into squares. Double the recipe for a large pan. These brownies will keep in the refrigerator for 4 weeks or more.

∾ Elaina

CHOCOLATE SUGAR-FREE PIE

Crust

RAW

- 3 cups walnuts, soaked 8 or more hours
- 1/2 cup ground dry chia seeds
- 1/2 cup carob powder
- 10 drops almond essence
- 1/2 cup shaved or shredded cacao butter (do not melt)
- 1/4 teaspoon salt
- 2/3 cup Irish Moss Paste (you will need 1 cup for the filling as well; see pp. 71–72)
- 1/2 cup Lakanto sugar or Erythritol or Xylitol to taste

Purée all the ingredients in a food processor until mixed well. Press into a 9-inch pie plate, covering the sides and bottom of the plate with dough.

Filling

- 1 cup Irish Moss Paste (1:1 ratio soaked moss to water; see pp. 71–72)
- 15 drops raspberry essence
- 6 drops vanilla extract
- 1/2 cup carob powder
- 1/2 cup cacao powder
- 2/3 cup shaved cacao butter
- 1 1/2 cups soaked walnuts
- 2 cups water
- 1/4 teaspoon liquid stevia
- 3/4 cup Lakanto, Erythritol, or Xylitol
- 1/2 teaspoon sea salt

Blend all the ingredients in a blender until smooth. Pour into the piecrust and let set for 1–2 hours in the refrigerator. Top with Sky High Whip.

Topping: Sky High Whip

> ¹/₄ cup soaked Irish moss (measure after soaking in cold water for 3+ hours)
> 1 cup water

Blend moss and water until smooth before adding:

> 1³/₄ cups water
> ³/₄ cup Lakanto sugar-free sweetener or Erythritol
> ³/₄ cup coconut oil
> 3 tablespoons powdered soy lecithin
> 1¹/₂ cups hempseeds or soaked and rinsed walnuts
> 15 drops vanilla extract essence or 1 tablespoon vanilla extract

Blend all the ingredients in a blender until smooth. Drop or pipe the whip onto pies and puddings with a pastry bag as desired. This topping will last for 1 week in the refrigerator.

∿ *Elaina*

CHOCO-CHIA-CINNAMON COOKIES

1/2 cup chia seeds, ground

2 cups dried, shredded coconut, powdered

1/2 cup carob powder

1/2 cup cacao powder

1/2 cup powdered Lakanto or coconut palm sugar (for sweeter cookies add 1/2 cup more sweetener)

10 drops vanilla essence

10 drops cherry essence

1/4 teaspoon liquid stevia

1 1/2 cups Irish Moss Paste (see pp. 71–72)

2 tablespoons coconut palm sugar

2 tablespoons organic peanut butter

2 tablespoons cacao butter

2 tablespoons powdered soy lecithin

1/2 teaspoon ground, dried orange peel

1 teaspoon cinnamon

1/4 teaspoon Himalayan salt

2 dashes nutmeg

Dash of cayenne

Grind the chia and dried coconut in a blender or coffee grinder until they are powdered. Put the chia, coconut, and the remaining ingredients in a food processor and purée everything until smooth. Roll into balls and flatten into cookies. Dehydrate at 115° until crunchy, or skip dehydrating them and eat as is.

∾ *Elaina*

COCONUT RASPBERRY YOGURT

6 young Thai coconuts (yields approximately 3 cups coconut
    meat and 7 cups water)
2–3 capsules probiotic powder
3 pints of fresh raspberries

Cut open the coconuts and scoop out the coconut meat to get approximately 3 cups. Blend the coconut meat with about 7 cups young coconut water until smooth and creamy. Pour the contents of your blender into a clean glass jar and mix in the contents of 2–3 capsules of your favorite probiotic powder. Place the jar in a warm place in your kitchen and cover with a clean towel. Leave for 6–10 hours.

You know the yogurt is ready when it has a fluffy consistency. It will keep in the refrigerator for at least a week. The color of your yogurt should be white. If it turns pink, discard it.

For one serving, pour 2 cups coconut yogurt in a bowl and add ½ pint fresh raspberries.   ■ SERVES 5

∾ *Victoria*

RAINBOW GREEN PUDDING

RAW

½ bunch kale, stems removed
1 cup strawberries
1 cup blueberries
1 mango, peeled and seeded
4 dates, pitted
5 sprigs mint
4 cups water
5 tablespoons chia seeds

Blend the ingredients except the chia seeds together well in a blender, using a tamper if needed. Add the chia seeds last, blend until smooth, and serve immediately. Pour the pudding into a nice glass and decorate with a slice of strawberry and a mint leaf. ■ **SERVES 4**

෴ *Victoria*

CHIA NETTLE PUDDING

3 cups stinging nettles (to avoid stinging during preparation,
   use gloves or a plastic bag)
2 cups strawberries
2 cups apple juice
5 tablespoons chia seeds

Blend the stinging nettles, strawberries, and apple juice together in a blender, using a tamper if needed. Add the chia seeds last, blend until smooth, and serve immediately, before the pudding solidifies. Pour into a nice glass and decorate with a slice of strawberry. ▪ **SERVES 3**

∽ *Victoria*

PAPAYA PUDDING

RAW

1 cup sunflower sprouts
1 small papaya, peeled and seeded

For a thicker consistency, blend these ingredients in a high-speed blender without adding water. Use a tamper if needed. Pour into nice glasses and decorate with a slice of fruit.

■ SERVES 2

~ *Victoria*

DRINKS

OMEGA-3 SEED MILK

RAW

1 cup walnuts, flaxseeds, or hempseeds, soaked for 4 hours

4 cups water

Stevia to taste

1/4 teaspoon sea salt

1 tablespoon Irish Moss Paste for texture (see pp. 71–72)
   (optional)

Rinse the seeds well and drain. Blend with the water until smooth (30 seconds). Strain through a nut milk bag. Blend in a few drops of stevia to taste. Add the sea salt. Try vanilla or toffee flavor, and add Irish Moss Paste if desired. You can refrigerate the milk in a glass jar for up to 5 days.

Store the seed or nut pulp in a ziplock bag laid flat in the freezer to use for cakes or bread later, but not longer than a month.

~ *Elaina*

BEST GREEN JUICE COMBO EVER MADE

RAW

4 stalks celery, chopped

2 cups spinach

$1/4$ bunch parsley

$1/4$ bunch cilantro

2 apples, peeled and chopped

1 cucumber, cut into large cubes

$1/4$ lemon, without peel

Juice all the ingredients in a juicer. Drink immediately.

■ YIELDS 1 QUART

∿ *Valya*

ELAINA'S POST-RUN SMOOTHIE

After running an hour or more, I really need to refuel quickly for optimal recovery and long-term strength. Here is my favorite smoothie after a run:

RAW

1 ripe banana

1 cup strawberries or other berry

2 large handfuls spinach, kale, or parsley

2 heaping tablespoons hemp protein powder

1 scoop L-glutamine (supplement for muscle recovery)

2 teaspoons powdered soy lecithin (for brain power and creaminess)

1 heaping tablespoon soaked chia seeds (see p. 84)

1 tablespoon Vitamineral Green powder

Few drops liquid stevia

Blend until smooth and creamy. Pour into a quart-size mason jar and drink over the next hour. ■ YIELDS ABOUT 1 QUART

∾ *Elaina*

CHIA MACA SHAKE

RAW

2 cups hempseed, walnut, or flaxseed milk
$^1/_4$ cup soaked chia seeds (see p. 84)
2 tablespoons ground flax meal
2–3 tablespoons maca powder
1–2 tablespoons powdered soy lecithin
4 drops vanilla essence or 1 vanilla bean
1 scoop probiotic powder or the contents of 1–2 probiotic
    capsules
Sweetener of choice: 6 drops stevia (best) or 2–4 tablespoons
    honey or maple syrup
$^3/_4$ cup ice cubes if desired

Blend until smooth. You can double or triple the recipe to make enough to last for the next couple days.

Green Chia Shake Variation

Eliminate ½ the maca and add 1 tablespoon green powder of your choice.

For variety, play around with different extracts like banana, coconut, maple, coffee, chai, etc.

$\sim$ *Elaina*

OMEGA-3 GREEN SMOOTHIE

RAW

4 cups purslane, leaves and stems

1 ripe mango, peeled and seeded

1 cup strawberries

4 cups water

1 tablespoon chia seeds

Blend well and serve.　　　　　　　　■ SERVES 5

∾ *Victoria*

FAST GREEN SMOOTHIE

RAW

1 bunch chard, stems removed

2 ripe mangoes, peeled and seeded

4 cups water

Combine the ingredients in a blender until smooth and serve.

■ YIELDS 1 QUART

∾ *Victoria*

PEAR-FECT SMOOTHIE

RAW

1 bunch curly kale

2 pears, chopped

2 bananas, peeled

2 sprigs fresh mint

4 cups water

Combine the ingredients in a blender until smooth and serve. Pour into a nice glass and decorate with a mint leaf. ■ SERVES 3

∽ *Victoria*

LETTUCE DRINK TO YOUR HEALTH

RAW

½ bunch red leaf lettuce
½ bunch oak leaf lettuce
1 cup strawberries
2 bananas, sliced
1 apple, chopped
4 cups water

Combine the ingredients in a blender until smooth and serve.
Pour into a nice glass and decorate with a slice of strawberry.

■ **SERVES 3**

∽ *Victoria*

DOCTOR GREEN

1 bunch fresh parsley
1 peeled cucumber
1 Fuji apple, chopped
1 ripe banana, peeled
1 thumb-size leaf aloe vera with skin from live plant
3 cups water

Combine the ingredients in a blender until smooth. Pour into a nice glass and decorate with thin slices of cucumber.

■ SERVES 3

∽ *Victoria*

SUPER GREEN SMOOTHIE

RAW

1 bunch chard, stems removed
1 large red bell pepper, without stem, but with seeds
2 cups water

Blend the ingredients in a blender until smooth. Pour into nice glasses and serve. ■ **SERVES 2**

∽ *Victoria*

GREEN SMOOTHIE FOR THYROID SUPPORT

RAW

1 bunch chard, stems removed

1 ripe mango, peeled and seeded

1 cup strawberries

2 tablespoons kelp, granulated or powder

4 cups water

Blend well and serve.   ■ YIELDS 1 QUART

∾ *Victoria*

GRASSHOPPER ON A BLUEBERRY

RAW

1 cup wheatgrass
1 cup spinach
1 cup blueberries
2 apples, chopped
1-inch piece ginger
1 banana
4 cups water

Blend well. Pour into a nice glass and decorate with several thin slices of spinach.   ■ SERVES 4

෴ *Victoria*

ACKNOWLEDGMENTS

We greatly appreciate our friends who volunteered to spend many hours editing our manuscript: Aletha Nowitzky, Vanessa Nowitzky, and Ines Compton.

We thank Valya Boutenko for graciously sharing her recipes for this book.

INDEX

Almonds
  ratio of omega-3s to omega-6s, 13
  Thai Broccoli with Almond Chile
    Sauce and Root Rice, 110–11
alpha-linolenic acid (ALA), 10
Anderson, Richard, 23
animal products, consuming, 8–9
animals, their consumption of raw
  foods, 5
appetizers, antipasti, and finger
  foods
  Avocado Nori Rolls, 49–50
  Cheeze Whip, 43
  Hemp Crostini, 42
  Marinated Baby Vegetables, Fresh
    Citrus Olives, Pickled Garlic
    and Sweet Peppers, 46–48
  Merlot Pickled Onions, 45
  Valya's Salsa, 44
  Walnut Falafel with Mint Tabouli
    and Hemp Tzatziki, 40–41
apples
  Fennel, Apple, and Arugula
    with Sunflower Sprouts and
    Mandarin Vinaigrette, 55
  Grasshopper on a Blueberry, 145
  Happy Colon Sorbet, 122
  Hemp Crostini, 42
  ratio of omega-3s to omega-6s, 17
arugula
  Arugula Salad, 58
  Fennel, Apple, and Arugula

  with Sunflower Sprouts and
    Mandarin Vinaigrette, 55
  ratio of omega-3s to omega-6s, 16
  Zucchini Pasta with Arugula-Pesto
    Sauce, 104
avocado
  Avocado Crème, 107
  Avocado Nori Rolls, 49–50
  Marinated Chard and Kale Salad,
    56–57
  ratio of omega-3s to omega-6s, 12
  Trio of Cabbages with Hemp,
    Avocado, and Cilantro, 54

Bananas
  ratio of omega-3s to omega-6s, 17
  See also smoothie and sorbet
    recipes
beans, green, ratio of omega-3s to
  omega-6s, 15
beans, red
  Chipotle Tostadas, 101
  Fat-Free Chipotle Red Beans, 115
beets
  Beet Salad, 61
  Marinated Baby Vegetables, 46
  Quick Borscht, 88
Bell Pepper Salad, 65
berries
  Chia Nettle Pudding, 130
  Grasshopper on a Blueberry, 145
  Rainbow Green Pudding, 129

berries *(continued)*
  See also smoothie recipes
Best Green Juice Combo Ever Made,
  135
Black Forest Carob Brownies, 124
Borscht, Quick, 88
breads
  Brown Walnut Bread, 94
  See also crackers and chips
broccoli
  Marinated Tender Broccoli and
    Zucchini, 117
  Thai Broccoli with Almond Chile
    Sauce and Root Rice, 110–11
Brown Rice, Fire-Roasted Tomato
  Lentil Chile with Avocado
  Crème and, 106–7
Brown Walnut Bread, 94
Butternut Squash Soup, 79

Cabbage
  Purple Salad, 53
  Trio of Cabbages with Hemp,
    Avocado, and Cilantro, 54
Caesar Salad, 52
calorie sources on the raw foods diet,
  20–21
Candied Walnuts, 60
canola oil, ratio of omega-3s to
  omega-6s, 11
Caramelized Shallots, 59–60
carob
  Black Forest Carob Brownies,
    124
  Choco-Chia-Cinnamon Cookies,
    127
  Chocolate Sugar-Free Pie, 125–26
carrots
  Marinated Baby Vegetables, 46
  ratio of omega-3s to omega-6s, 17
cashews, ratio of omega-3s to
  omega-6s, 13
celery
  Celery Soup, 85
  Italian Soup, 82
  Mushroom-Potato Soup, 86
Cheeze Whip, 43

chia seeds
  Brown Walnut Bread, 94
  Chia Maca Shake, 137
  Chia Nettle Pudding, 130
  Choco-Chia-Cinnamon Cookies,
    127
  Chocolate Sugar-Free Pie, 125–26
  Crunchy Chia Crisps, 97–98
  Omega-3 Birdseed Flax Crackers,
    96
  ratio of omega-3s to omega-6s, 12
  soaked, 84
chickpeas, ratio of omega-3s to
  omega-6s, 15
Chile, Fire-Roasted Tomato Lentil
  with Avocado Crème and
  Brown Rice, 106–7
Chipotle Tostadas, 101
chips. *See* crackers and chips
chocolate
  Choco-Chia-Cinnamon Cookies,
    127
  Chocolate Sugar-Free Pie, 125–26
cilantro
  Cilantro-Walnut Crackers or Dip,
    95
  Creamy Cilantro Soup, 84
  Trio of Cabbages with Hemp,
    Avocado, and Cilantro, 54
citrus fruits
  Fresh Citrus Olives, 47
  Pink Grapefruit Cream Sorbet
    Decadence, 123
  Valya's Silly-Yum Sorbet, 121
cocoa butter, ratio of omega-3s to
  omega-6s, 12
coconut meat, raw
  Choco-Chia-Cinnamon Cookies,
    127
  Coconut Raspberry Yogurt, 128
  Miso Broth with Coconut Soba, 91
  ratio of omega-3s to omega-6s, 12
coconut oil, ratio of omega-3s to
  omega-6s, 12
cooked food *vs.* raw food
  Boutenko on, 4–5, 21–22
  Love on, 23–27, 29

Sarno on, 32–36
cookies. *See* desserts
corn
    Chipotle Tostadas, 101
    corn oil, ratio of omega-3s to
      omega-6s, 11
    Quinoa Salad, 66
crackers and chips
    Cilantro-Walnut Crackers or Dip,
      95
    Crunchy Chia Crisps, 97–98
    Kale Chips, 99–100
    Omega-3 Birdseed Flax Crackers,
      96
Creamy Cilantro Soup, 84
Crunchy Chia Crisps, 97–98

Dandelion greens, ratio of omega-3s
    to omega-6s, 16
desserts
    Black Forest Carob Brownies, 124
    Chia Nettle Pudding, 130
    Choco-Chia-Cinnamon Cookies,
      127
    Chocolate Sugar-Free Pie, 125–26
    Coconut Raspberry Yogurt, 128
    Happy Colon Sorbet, 122
    Low-Glycemic Omega-3 Coffee
      "Ice Cream," 120
    Pink Grapefruit Cream Sorbet
      Decadence, 123
    Rainbow Green Pudding, 129
    Sky High Whip, 126
    Valya's Silly-Yum Sorbet, 121
disease
    and essential fatty acids balance,
      9–10
    and food choices, 29
DNA manipulation of seeds, 8
Doctor Green (smoothie), 142
dressings and marinades
    for Beet Salad, 61
    for Caesar Salad, 52
    Fresh Vegan Mayo, 71–72
    Italian Marinade, 46
    Mandarin Vinaigrette, 70
    Marinade for Chard and Kale

    Salad, 56–57
    Ranch Dressing, 74
    Raspberry Vinaigrette, 59
    Red Bell Pepper Dressing, 75
    Sweet Miso-Ginger Dressing, 67
    Tomato-Dill Dressing, 73
drinks
    Best Green Juice Combo Ever
      Made, 135
    Chia Maca Shake, 137
    Doctor Green, 142
    Grasshopper on a Blueberry, 145
    Lettuce Drink to Your Health, 141
    Omega-3 Green Smoothie, 138
    Omega-3 Seed Milk, 134
    Pear-Fect Smoothie, 140
    Super Green Smoothie, 143

Eicosapentaenoic acid (EPA), 10
Elaina's Post-Run Smoothie, 136
energy bars, 19
entrées
    Fat-Free Chipotle Red Beans, 115
    Fire-Roasted Tomato Lentil Chile
      with Avocado Crème and
      Brown Rice, 106–7
    Lentils in Heaven, 105
    Mac 'n' Cheeze, 116
    Marinated Tender Broccoli and
      Zucchini, 117
    Marinated Vegetable Lasagna,
      112–13
    Steamed Veggies, 114
    Thai Broccoli with Almond Chile
      Sauce and Root Rice, 110–11
    Wild Mushroom Croquettes with
      Rustic Puttanesca, 108–9
    Zucchini Pasta with Arugula-Pesto
      Sauce, 104
essential fatty acids. *See* omega-3
    fatty acids

Fast Green Smoothie, 139
Fat-Free Chipotle Red Beans, 115
Fennel, Apple, and Arugula with
    Sunflower Sprouts and
    Mandarin Vinaigrette, 55

Field Greens with Caramelized
    Shallots, Candied Walnuts, and
    Raspberry Vinaigrette, 59–60
filberts, ratio of omega-3s to
    omega-6s, 14
finger foods. *See* appetizers, antipasti,
    and finger foods
Fire-Roasted Tomato Lentil Chile
    with Avocado Crème and
    Brown Rice, 106–7
fish consumption, 9
flaxseeds
    Brown Walnut Bread, 94
    Chia Maca Shake, 137
    flaxseed oil, ratio of omega-3s to
        omega-6s, 10
    Hemp Crostini, 42
    Omega-3 Birdseed Flax Crackers,
        96
    Omega-3 Seed Milk, 134
    ratio of omega-3s to omega-6s, 12
food pyramids, Boutenko's, 22
fractionated foods, 36
Fresh Citrus Olives, 47
Fresh Vegan Mayo, 71–72

Garden Minestrone with Wild Rice
    and Sage Pesto, 89–90
Garlic, Pickled and Sweet Peppers,
    47–48
gourmet raw foods, 26–27, 33
Grasshopper on a Blueberry, 145
green peas, ratio of omega-3s to
    omega-6s, 15
green smoothies, 6–7
    Chia Maca Shake, green variation,
        137
    Doctor Green, 142
    Elaina's Post-Run Smoothie, 136
    Fast Green Smoothie, 139
    Grasshopper on a Blueberry, 145
    Green Smoothie for Thyroid
        Support, 144
    Lettuce Drink to Your Health, 141
    Omega-3 Green Smoothie, 138
    Pear-Fect Smoothie, 140
    Super Green Smoothie, 143

Happy Colon Sorbet, 122
hazelnuts, ratio of omega-3s to
    omega-6s, 14
healing and detoxing food pyramid,
    22
"Health Starts Here" program, 36
hempseeds
    Cheeze Whip, 43
    Chia Maca Shake, 137
    Hemp Crostini, 42
    hempseed oil, ratio of omega-3s to
        omega-6s, 11
    Hemp Tzatziki, 41
    Omega-3 Birdseed Flax Crackers,
        96
    Omega-3 Seed Milk, 134
    Ranch Dressing, 74
    Ranch Kale Chips, 99–100
    ratio of omega-3s to omega-6s, 12
    Trio of Cabbages with Hemp,
        Avocado, and Cilantro, 54
high-raw diet, 19, 21, 23, 25, 27, 30
Howell, Edward, 3

"Ice Cream," Low-Glycemic
    Omega-3 Coffee, 120
Irish Moss Paste, 71–72
Italian Marinade, 46
Italian Soup, 82

Kale
    Kale Chips, 99–100
    Marinated Chard and Kale Salad,
        56–57
    Pear-Fect Smoothie, 140
    Rainbow Green Pudding, 129
    Yellow Split Pea Soup with
        Smoked Dulse and Kale, 92
kidney beans, ratio of omega-3s to
    omega-6s, 15

Lambsquarters
    Wild Weeds Soup, 80
Lasagna, Marinated Vegetable, 112–13
lentils
    Fire-Roasted Tomato Lentil Chile
        with Avocado Crème and

Brown Rice, 106–7
Lentils in Heaven, 105
ratio of omega-3s to omega-6s, 15
Vegetable Soup with Lentils, 87
lettuce
    cos or romaine, ratio of omega-3s
        to omega-6s, 16
    Lettuce Drink to Your Health, 141
    raw green-leaf, ratio of omega-3s
        to omega-6s, 16
Living Light Culinary Arts Institute,
    31
Low-Glycemic Omega-3 Coffee "Ice
    Cream," 120

Maca
    Chia Maca Shake, 137
macadamia nuts, ratio of omega-3s
    to omega-6s, 13
Mac 'n' Cheeze, 116
Mandarin Vinaigrette, 70
marinades
    Italian Marinade, 46
    Marinated Baby Vegetables, Fresh
        Citrus Olives, Pickled Garlic
        and Sweet Peppers, 46–48
    Marinated Chard and Kale Salad,
        56–57
    Marinated Tender Broccoli and
        Zucchini, 117
    Marinated Vegetable Lasagna,
        112–13
    See also dressings and marinades
Mayo, Fresh Vegan, 71–72
meat consumption, 8–9
Merlot Pickled Onions, 45
milks. See drinks
Mint Tabouli and Hemp Tzatziki,
    40–41
miso
    Miso Broth with Coconut Soba, 91
    Miso-Ginger dressing, 67
    Spicy Miso Paste, 49–50
mushrooms
    Mushroom-Potato Soup, 86
    Wild Mushroom Croquettes with
        Rustic Puttanesca, 108–9

mustard greens
    Spicy Green Soup, 78
    Wild Weeds Soup, 80

Nettles, stinging. See stinging nettles
Noodle Salad with Sweet Miso-
    Ginger Dressing, 67
nuts
    as calorie source, changing
        paradigm of, 17–18, 19, 20–21
    new raw foodists and, 26
    See also specific nuts

Oats, ratio of omega-3s to
    omega-6s, 14
olives
    Arugula Salad, 58
    Fresh Citrus Olives, 47
    olive oil, ratio of omega-3s to
        omega-6s, 11
Omega-3 Birdseed Flax Crackers, 96
omega-3 fatty acids
    deficiency of, Boutenko on, 7–10
    in foods, ratio of omega-3 to
        omega-6, 10–17
    incorporating into recipes, Love
        on, 28
    and the raw food paradigm,
        transformation of, 17–19
Omega-3 Green Smoothie, 138
Omega-3 Seed Milk, 134
omega-6 fatty acids, 8
onions
    Caramelized Shallots, 59–60
    Marinated Chard and Kale Salad,
        56
    Merlot Pickled Onions, 45
    Valya's Salsa, 44
    Vegetable Soup with Lentils, 87

Papaya Pudding, 131
parsley
    Doctor Green (smoothie), 142
    Fresh Mint Tabouli, 40–51
parsnips
    Root Rice: Parsnip and Sesame,
        110–11

peanuts, ratio of omega-3s to
    omega-6s, 14
pears
    Fennel, Apple, and Arugula
        with Sunflower Sprouts and
        Mandarin Vinaigrette, 55
    Hemp Crostini, 42
    Pear-Fect Smoothie, 140
peas
    Arugula Salad, 58
    Simply Delicious Pea Soup, 81
    See also split peas
pecans, ratio of omega-3s to
    omega-6s, 14
peppers
    Bell Pepper Salad, 65
    Pickled Garlic and Sweet Peppers,
        47–48
    Red Bell Marinara, 112
    Red Bell Pepper Dressing, 75
    Super Green Smoothie, 143
Pesto, Sage, 90
Pickled Garlic and Sweet Peppers,
    47–48
pine nuts, ratio of omega-3s to
    omega-6s, 14
Pink Grapefruit Cream Sorbet
    Decadence, 123
potatoes
    Lentils in Heaven, 105
    Mushroom-Potato Soup, 86
    Sweet Potato Weight-Loss Salad,
        62
    Vegetable Soup with Lentils, 87
produce quality, and raw foods
    success, 18
pumpkin seeds, ratio of omega-3s to
    omega-6s, 13
Purple Salad, 53
purslane, 10
    Omega-3 Green Smoothie, 138
    Wild Weeds Soup, 80
pyramid, food, 22

Quick Borscht, 88
quinoa
    Quinoa Salad, 66
    ratio of omega-3s to omega-6s, 15

Rainbow Green Pudding, 129
Ranch Dressing, 74
Ranch Kale Chips, 99–100
rancidity, omega-3 oils and, 19
Raspberry Vinaigrette, 59
raw food vs. cooked food
    Boutenko on, 4–5
    Love on, 23–27, 29
    Sarno on, 32–36
Red Bell Marinara, 112
Red Bell Pepper Dressing, 75
rice
    Brown, Fire-Roasted Tomato
        Lentil Chile with Avocado
        Crème and, 106–7
    Root Rice, 110–11
    wild rice sprouts, 89–90
Ricotta, 112
Righteous Salad, 64
Root Rice: Parsnip and Sesame,
    110–11
Rosemary Rain Soup, 83
Rustic Puttanesca, 109
rye, ratio of omega-3s to omega-6s,
    14

Safflower oil, ratio of omega-3s to
    omega-6s, 11
Sage Pesto, 90
salads
    Arugula Salad, 58
    Beet Salad, 61
    Bell Pepper Salad, 65
    Caesar Salad, 52
    Fennel, Apple, and Arugula
        with Sunflower Sprouts and
        Mandarin Vinaigrette, 55
    Field Greens with Caramelized
        Shallots, Candied Walnuts, and
        Raspberry Vinaigrette, 59–60
    Marinated Chard and Kale Salad,
        56–57
    Noodle Salad with Sweet Miso-
        Ginger Dressing, 67
    Purple Salad, 53
    Quinoa Salad, 66
    Righteous Salad, 64
    Sprout Salad, 63

Sweet Potato Weight-Loss Salad,
62
Trio of Cabbages with Hemp,
Avocado, and Cilantro, 54
sauces
Almond Chile Sauce, 110
Arugula-Pesto Sauce, 104
Red Bell Marinara, 112
Rustic Puttanesca, 109
See also dressings and marinades
seaweed
Avocado Nori Rolls, 49–50
Yellow Split Pea Soup with
Smoked Dulse and Kale, 92
seeds, DNA manipulation of, 8
sesame seeds
ratio of omega-3s to omega-6s, 13
sesame oil, ratio of omega-3s to
omega-6s, 11
Walnut Falafel, 40
Shallots, Caramelized, 59–60
Simply Delicious Pea Soup, 81
Sky High Whip, 126
smoothies, green. See green
smoothies
Soaked Chia Seeds, 84
sorbet. See desserts
Soria, Cherie, 31
soups
Butternut Squash Soup, 79
Celery Soup, 85
Creamy Cilantro Soup, 84
Garden Minestrone with Wild
Rice and Sage Pesto, 89–90
Italian Soup, 82
Miso Broth with Coconut Soba, 91
Mushroom-Potato Soup, 86
Quick Borscht, 88
Rosemary Rain Soup, 83
Simply Delicious Pea Soup, 81
Spicy Green Soup, 78
Vegetable Soup with Lentils, 87
Wild Weeds Soup, 80
Yellow Split Pea Soup with
Smoked Dulse and Kale, 92
Spicy Miso Paste, 49–50
spinach
Grasshopper on a Blueberry, 145

Italian Soup, 82
ratio of omega-3s to omega-6s, 16
spiritual attitude re: food-taking,
25–26
split peas
Yellow Split Pea Soup with
Smoked Dulse and Kale, 92
sprouts
Fennel, Apple, and Arugula
with Sunflower Sprouts and
Mandarin Vinaigrette, 55
Papaya Pudding, 131
red bean sprouts, 115
Sprout Salad, 63
sushi, 49
wild rice sprouts, 89–90
squash
Butternut Squash Soup, 79
Mac 'n' Cheeze, 116
Marinated Tender Broccoli and
Zucchini, 117
Zucchini Pasta with Arugula-Pesto
Sauce, 104
Steamed Veggies, 114
stinging nettles
Chia Nettle Pudding, 130
Spicy Green Soup, 78
strawberries
ratio of omega-3s to omega-6s,
17
See also smoothie recipes
sugar snap peas, ratio of omega-3s to
omega-6s, 16
sunflower seeds
Fennel, Apple, and Arugula
with Sunflower Sprouts and
Mandarin Vinaigrette, 55
ratio of omega-3s to omega-6s,
13
sprouts, Papaya Pudding, 131
sunflower oil, ratio of omega-3s to
omega-6s, 11
Super Green Smoothie, 143
sushi, Avocado Nori Rolls, 49–50
sustainable diet, 21–22, 32–33, 35
Sweet Miso-Ginger Dressing, 67
Sweet Potato Weight-Loss Salad,
62

Swiss chard
    Fast Green Smoothie, 139
    Green Smoothie for Thyroid
        Support, 144
    Marinated Chard and Kale Salad,
        56–57
    Super Green Smoothie, 143
symptoms experienced on raw foods
    diet, 5, 7

Tabouli, Fresh Mint, 40–41
Thai Broccoli with Almond Chile
        Sauce and Root Rice, 110–11
tilapia, farmed, 9
Tomato-Dill Kale Chips, 99–100
tomatoes
    Celery Soup, 85
    Tomato-Dill Dressing, 73
    Tomato-Dill Kale Chips, 99–100
    Valya's Salsa, 44
Tostadas, Chipotle, 101
triglyceride levels, 34–35
Trio of Cabbages with Hemp,
        Avocado, and Cilantro, 54

Valya's Salsa, 44
Valya's Silly-Yum Sorbet, 121
vegan diet, 34
vegetables, mixed
    Marinated Baby Vegetables, Fresh
        Citrus Olives, Pickled Garlic
        and Sweet Peppers, 46–48
    Marinated Vegetable Lasagna,
        112–13
    Steamed Veggies, 114
    Vegetable Soup with Lentils, 87
    See also specific vegetables

Walnuts
    Black Forest Carob Brownies, 124

Brown Walnut Bread, 94
Candied Walnuts, 60
Cheeze Whip, 43
Chia Maca Shake, 137
Chocolate Sugar-Free Pie,
        125–26
Cilantro-Walnut Crackers or Dip,
        95
Omega-3 Seed Milk, 134
Ranch Dressing, 74
Ranch Kale Chips, 99–100
ratio of omega-3s to omega-6s,
        13
Ricotta, 112
Walnut Falafel with Mint Tabouli
        and Hemp Tzatziki, 40–41
Wild Mushroom Croquettes with
        Rustic Puttanesca, 108–9
warm climates, raw foods success
        and, 18
wheat, ratio of omega-3s to
        omega-6s, 14
wheatgrass
    Grasshopper on a Blueberry,
        145
Whole Foods Market, 36
Wild Mushroom Croquettes with
        Rustic Puttanesca, 108–9
wild rice, softening, 89–90
Wild Weeds Soup, 80

Yellow Split Pea Soup with Smoked
        Dulse and Kale, 92

Zucchini
    Mac 'n' Cheeze, 116
    Marinated Baby Vegetables, 46
    Marinated Tender Broccoli and
        Zucchini, 117
    Zucchini Pasta with Arugula-Pesto
        Sauce, 104

ABOUT THE AUTHORS

 Victoria Boutenko is the award-winning author of *Green for Life, Raw Family: A True Story of Awakening, 12 Steps to Raw Foods, Green Smoothie Revolution,* and *Raw Family Signature Dishes.* A raw gourmet chef, teacher, inventor, researcher, and artist, she has helped millions of people discover green smoothies and raw food. To learn more about her teachings, visit www.rawfamily.com.

 Elaina Love is an instructor at the renowned Living Light Culinary Arts Institute and has been teaching raw food courses worldwide since 1998. Owner-director of the online raw food store and website Pure Joy Planet (www.purejoyplanet.com), she lives in Patagonia, Arizona.

 Chad Sarno is founder and director of Vital Creations (www.rawchef.com), an internationally renowned restaurant consultancy, personal chef and catering service, and food design firm. A former personal chef to Woody Harrelson, he joined Whole Foods in 2009 to help launch the company's Healthy Eating Initiative. He lives in Austin, Texas.